THE
PREGNANCY
POCKET BIBLE

THE
PREGNANCY
POCKET BIBLE

HOLLIE SMITH

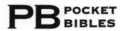

This edition first published in Great Britain 2009 by
Crimson Publishing, a division of Crimson Business Ltd
Westminster House
Kew Road
Richmond
Surrey
TW9 2ND

A catalogue record for this book is available from the British Library.

ISBN 978–1–907087–07–3

Typeset by RefineCatch Ltd, Bungay, Suffolk
Printed and bound by LegoPrint SpA, Trento

CONTENTS

INTRODUCTION

Pregnancy is one of the biggest, if not *the* biggest, events of your life. For a first-time mother-to-be, or even the seasoned pro, pregnancy can seem utterly daunting. You'll have information thrown at you from all sides – from your mother, friends, partner, antenatal classmates, doctors and midwives. All of this can be hard to digest, let alone remember when you need it.

The Pregnancy Pocket Bible includes all the information and advice you could want and need during your pregnancy – so you can look up anything you're not sure of at once, and don't have to go routing through piles of notes and leaflets.

Pregnancy is an amazing, life-changing experience – and having a baby growing inside of you seems like a miracle. Throughout, we have included many weird and wonderful facts to show you just how special this time of your life is. We've also included lots of tips and advice to help your pregnancy go as smoothly as possible.

The most important thing during pregnancy is to enjoy it. And get ready for what the future holds.

> 'A mother's joy begins when new life is stirring inside . . .
> when a tiny heartbeat is heard for the very first time, and a
> playful kick reminds her that she is never alone.'
>
> *Author unknown*

Author's Note

I have referred to the baby as a boy throughout, and to midwives as female and doctors as male. This is only to make for ease of reading.

CONGRATULATIONS, YOU'RE PREGNANT!

You're having a baby. Whether you've been trying for a while, or whether it's a surprise to you, one thing's for sure: the next nine months are likely to be challenging, exciting, and scary in equal measure.

20 GREAT THINGS ABOUT BEING PREGNANT

1. It can feel amazing to have created a new life – with your partner.

2. You get free dental care from now until your baby is one year old.

3. It's an excuse to pamper yourself – you won't have time when your baby arrives!

4. You can take a nap when you feel like it, and not feel guilty

5. Feeling your baby's first kick – it is truly miraculous.

6. People give up their seat in public places and open doors for you (theoretically).

7. The 'glow' – once you get over the morning sickness, you'll blossom as your hair gets shinier and your skin is rosy.

8. You'll never be on your own or lonely for nine months, and will always have someone to talk to.

9. You won't get your period for slightly more than nine months.

10. You get to eat more (but be careful of eating for two!).

11. If you're pregnant during winter, your baby will help keep you warm.

12. Relishing the first few weeks when you and your partner have an amazing secret.

13. Seeing the looks on your friends' and family's faces when you tell them your news.

14. Dreaming of the future – what your baby will look like, what personality they'll have, what their career will be – dream big!

15. For the less well endowed, this is your chance to have a cleavage!

16. Choosing baby clothes. They are always cute.

17. Reading about how your baby grows – and being astounded by the facts.

18. It is the best reason and incentive you'll ever get to give up smoking.

19. Maternity leave – time to prepare yourself, and enjoy your baby when it comes.

20. Friendliness of everyone you meet. Goodwill increases ten-fold to a pregnant woman.

🍼 AMAZING PREGNANCY FACTS 🍼

- There are **600,000 babies born every year** in the UK.

- A baby is born somewhere in the world **every three seconds**.

- The **youngest person** ever to give birth is Lina Medina, a Peruvian girl from the Andean village of Ticrapo. She gave birth to a boy by Caesarean section on 14 May 1939 at the age of 5 years, 7 months and 21 days.

- The **world's youngest parents** were 8 and 9 years old and lived in China in 1910.

- The **heaviest baby** ever born was to Canadian Anna Bates in 1979.

- The **longest baby** ever born may be Charlie Stokes from Wiltshire. He was born in 2005 and weighed 15lbs 2oz and measured 69cm from rump to head.

- The **greatest number of children born** to one woman is 69. In the 1700s a woman from Russia had 16 sets of twins, seven sets of triplets and four sets of quadruplets.

- The world's **first pregnant man** was Thomas Beatie, who gave birth to Susan on 29 June 2008. After gender reassignment surgery, Beatie was legally male but kept his reproductive organs and had a natural birth. His second baby, a boy, was born in June 2009.

Pocket fact 🎲

Wilma Flintstone was the first animated character that was portrayed as pregnant. She was pictured during several episodes of season 3 leading up to the eventual birth of Pebbles.

DISCOVERING YOU'RE PREGNANT

🛒 SHALL I TELL EVERYONE? 🛒

It's traditional to keep it to yourself for a while to save you having to tell everyone should anything go wrong. The early months are the most risky. There are a few people you probably should tell first:

- the baby's father!

- prospective grandparents

- any close family you want to know.

Many couples choose to keep it to themselves while they get used to the idea and enjoy keeping their amazing secret.

After your 12-week scan, most people feel it's safe to tell everyone.

Pocket tip 🍼

You don't have to tell anyone at work for quite a long time yet. Technically you can keep it to yourself until up to 15 weeks before you're due, although your bump is likely to start showing at some point in the first trimester (the first three months), and it's advisable to tell work soonish, so you can sort out maternity cover.

👶 FIRST SIGNS OF PREGNANCY 👶

Right from the start, your body begins the first in a whole series of very normal and natural changes, as the new life inside you takes root.

Pocket fact 🎲

In Turkish tradition, a pregnant woman is not allowed to look at a monkey, chew gum, attend a funeral or eat fish.

Early signs of pregnancy include:

- tender, 'tingling' or slightly bigger breasts; darkening of the areola (the skin round the nipple)

- a heightened sense of smell or taste

- going off one or more foods or drinks, or craving something in particular. Some women say they have an odd 'metallic' taste in the mouth

- nausea – so-called 'morning sickness' can kick in within days of conception

- feeling weepy and sensitive

- exhaustion

- needing to urinate a lot

- a missed period (although you may still experience a little light bleeding, known as 'spotting', and this isn't necessarily anything to worry about – see p. 62).

Turn to p. 20 for a detailed explanation of what's happening to your body.

Pocket tip ☞

Remember that every pregnancy is unique – some women escape with a few niggling symptoms, others experience a whole catalogue of complaints.

👶 GETTING USED TO THE IDEA 👶

Of course, it's not just your body that's affected in the early days of pregnancy – your mind is, too. Having a baby is a big responsibility, and discovering you're pregnant is undoubtedly a life-changing moment.

- Emotionally, expect to feel anything from ecstatic to scared – or a combination.

- It's perfectly normal to feel a whole range of less than positive feelings, even if your pregnancy was something you planned.

- Don't feel bad if you don't feel that good about it at first. It's normal – most people need some time to get their head round the reality of being pregnant.

HIS REACTION

It's traditional for men to be a little freaked out by a positive result (regardless of the fact that they impregnated you quite knowingly), so all in all, the first few weeks of pregnancy can be a bit of an emotional rollercoaster for you both.

Remember not to get worried or upset if he seems scared at first – for many men it doesn't 'hit home' that they are actually having a baby until they see an ultrasound (seeing is believing).

Talk to each other and keep communicating about how you feel.

Pocket tip 🗭

Remember millions and millions of other people have become parents, and have had exactly the same feeling as you.

👶 GOING IT ALONE 👶

If you're on your own (or in an unstable relationship, and likely to be that way before very long), you may be feeling even more anxious about what the future holds. Draw on the support of anyone else around you who cares, or among your family and friends, so that you never have to go to a scan on your own and there'll always be someone on the end of a phone. There are also lots of organisations and websites that offer information, advice and friendship.

Pocket fact 🔡

Every pregnant woman is entitled to a Health in Pregnancy Grant. This one-off payment from the Government is available to all women who are 25 weeks pregnant or more. You can pick up a claim form from your midwife or doctor.

🛒 WORKING OUT YOUR DUE DATE 🛒

Your EDD is your estimated delivery date (sometimes also called estimated date of confinement, or just due date). Your GP or midwife will work it out for you at your first appointment, or if you can't wait, you can do the sums yourself:

• Count 40 weeks on from the first day of your last menstrual period (LMP), which is when pregnancy is considered to start. This calculation gives you a fair idea of when you're due, but it does assume your periods follow a regular 28-day cycle, which isn't the case for everyone.

If your periods are irregular, you'll be able to find out for sure when you have your first ultrasound scan and your baby's measurements will give an accurate idea of when you're due. If this differs from the LMP date you've already worked out, it will now be considered the one to go by.

Pocket fact 🎲
Fewer than 5% of babies arrive on their EDD.

'Pregnancy is a miracle, the height of creativity for any woman.'

Barbra Streisand

3

YOUR ANTENATAL CARE: A ROUGH GUIDE

🚼 YOUR ANTENATAL CARE 🚼

Systems of antenatal care vary around the country and even according to which specific clinic, surgery or hospital you attend. The care you're offered may also be influenced by choices you've made yourself, and any risk factors that may affect you.

- Responsibility for keeping an eye on you may be shared between your GP and midwife, and can be midwife-led or GP-led.

- If you have any complicating factors to your pregnancy, a hospital consultant obstetrician will take charge overall, perhaps even seeing you in person during check-ups.

- Some health authorities run what's called a domino scheme, where a whole team of community-based midwives look after you during your pregnancy, one of whom, in theory, will be with you during the birth, too.

Whatever system is offered to you should be explained by whoever you see first.

Pocket tip 🖎

If you have any questions about your antenatal care, ask. That's what the medical professionals are there for.

If you don't understand something, ask. Usually GPs and midwives are pretty good at explaining things in plain English, but there's no harm in double-checking you've understood.

🛒 YOUR FIRST CHECK-UP 🛒

This should take place as soon as possible after you know you're pregnant, some time before the 10th week of pregnancy, since some of the tests you'll be offered need to be carried out before then. During this initial check-up (often known as a booking appointment) you'll be given a lot of information, have to answer lots of questions, and will be asked to undergo a number of tests.

What to expect at your booking appointment

- You'll be asked lots of questions and may have to fill in lots of forms to help create a complete picture of your health (and your partner's), family history, work and lifestyle – all things that may in some way affect you, your pregnancy or your baby.

- You'll be asked about where you want to have your baby (see below).

- You'll be weighed, your height measured and your BMI (body mass index) calculated. Your midwife needs to know if you're significantly overweight or underweight, as these could prove complicating factors.

- You'll be asked for a urine sample (as you will on all subsequent check-ups). This can help doctors detect a number of potential problems.

- Your blood pressure will be taken – at this and every subsequent check-up. It's common for blood pressure to rise in pregnancy and it's important to keep tabs on it because if it gets too high, it's a sign of pre-eclampsia (see p. 56).

- You'll have a number of blood samples taken.

- You'll also be offered two tests, one early on and one later (at 28 weeks), to check for iron-deficiency anaemia.

- You'll be given lots of other information about looking after yourself and the baby, the further tests and scans (see below) that you'll be offered, and your choices regarding your antenatal care and the birth.

🛒 SUBSEQUENT APPOINTMENTS 🛒

These will be much shorter and will usually involve just urine and blood pressure checks. Regular checks on the baby will also be involved – your abdomen will be felt to check his position and growth, and his heartbeat monitored. It's a good time to ask any questions or voice any concerns you may have.

Pocket fact 🎲

The longest animal pregnancy is the Alpine Salamander of Southern Europe, which is pregnant for 38 months. Elephants are pregnant for 22 months. And possums have one of the shortest pregnancies at 16 days.

How frequent should appointments be?

According to official guidelines, antenatal appointments should take place every four weeks until you're 28 weeks pregnant, then every three weeks until 38 weeks.

You should then get one at 40 weeks and, after that, if you haven't yet given birth, you'll be seen at least weekly.

The National Institute for Healthy and Clinical Excellence (NICE) document called 'Routine antenatal care for healthy pregnant women' will let you know what you're entitled to. You can download it from the NICE website at www.nice.org.uk

---

🚼 CHECK-UPS IN THE 🚼 LAST TRIMESTER

You'll have more antenatal checks in your final trimester – it varies according to area, but in theory you should be seen at 28, 31, 34, 36, 38 and 40 weeks.

- Your midwife should measure your abdomen to make sure your baby's growing at roughly the expected rate.

- From about 36 weeks, she'll probably have a good feel each time to find out which way the baby is 'presenting', or lying.

- You'll also continue to have routine testing of your urine and blood pressure.

Pocket fact 🎲

Ultrasound scans often catch babies smiling weeks before they are born.

🍼 YOUR ANTENATAL NOTES 🍼

All pregnant women are given their own personal set of antenatal notes — you'll usually be asked to keep hold of them yourself in between appointments, so you'll need to take care of them and remember them at each appointment. These notes may also contain useful information such as telephone numbers for your doctor, midwife, clinic or maternity unit, and advice on what to do if anything concerns you.

🍼 ULTRASOUND SCANS 🍼

Scans allow the experts — and you — to get a glimpse of the life inside your womb by using sound waves.

According to guidelines from the National Institute for Health and Clinical Excellence (NICE), **you should be offered two routine ultrasound scans** during your pregnancy, including one at some point between 10 and 13 weeks, usually known as a dating scan.

3D scans

3D and 4D scans allow a really detailed look at a baby in the womb. You definitely won't get one of these on the NHS, so if you want one, contact a specialist clinic.

DATING SCAN

- A dating scan means you can confirm your EDD by taking the baby's measurements.

- It will reveal how many babies you've got in there!

- Depending on the policy of your hospital, you may also be offered nuchal translucency screening during this scan (see

'Pocket tip', p. 16). And generally speaking, most couples are glad of the reassurance that their baby is alive and kicking around now, having made it through the hairy weeks of the relatively high-risk first trimester.

> *Pocket tip* ☞
>
> *There are still a few places in the UK where dating scans are not offered routinely, and sometimes expectant couples who aren't offered a 12-week scan as a matter of course will choose to have one done privately for peace of mind, usually at a cost of around £100 to £150.*

SECOND SCAN

You will be offered a scan at around 18–20 weeks, by which time it's possible to see the baby in a lot more detail. This one is known as an anomaly, or mid-pregnancy, scan and is used to detect any abnormalities in the baby (although it's not guaranteed to pick up every potential problem) and to check all's well with his growth and position.

What happens at a scan?

- *Scans are completely painless and have no unpleasant side effects or consequences.*
- *You'll be asked to drink plenty of water and present yourself with a full bladder (it can help to push up your womb and so give a clearer picture).*
- *Gel is wiped across your naked tummy to help the probe glide across, and this is usually rather cold.*

- *Sonographers – the trained professionals who carry out scans – tend to work in silence, concentrating on seeking out all the baby's bits, and taking measurements. This can seem a little ominous, but it's normal.*
- *It's not always easy to make out the baby or its limbs – the sonographer will talk you through what they can see.*
- *Some hospitals will let you take away a photograph, usually for a small charge.*

Pocket tip 🗯

The website of the Fetal Anomaly Screening Programme (http://fetalanomaly.screening.nhs.uk/) is a good source of further information about scans.

🚼 BOY OR GIRL? 🚼

It's increasingly common to find out the baby's sex at the anomaly scan.

If you *do* want to know whether it's a girl or a boy, bear in mind that you may not be offered this information automatically, and might have to request it (ask at the beginning rather than the end of the scan, so there's time for the sonographer to look).

There are still some hospitals where the policy is not to let on, usually because they can't guarantee it will be accurate.

Remember, no one can give a 100% guarantee of an accurate answer to this question. Once in a while, an umbilical cord gets mistaken for a willy – and little Johnny turns out to be a Jane.

Pocket fact 🎲

Babies conceived during colder months have a slightly higher IQ than those conceived during warmer months.

OLD WIVES' TALES

Here are some ways of guessing the sex of your baby, to be taken with a pinch of salt . . .

Suspend a wedding ring on a string over the pregnant woman's hand. The direction it swings will determine the gender.

It's a boy if . . .

- You didn't experience morning sickness.
- Your extra weight is round your front.
- The bump is low.
- Your areola (area around your nipples) has gone very dark.
- Your feet are cold a lot.
- You crave protein.
- The father is gaining weight too.
- Add your age at the time of conception to the number of the month you conceived. If the amount is even, it's a boy.

It's a girl if . . .

- You experienced morning sickness.
- Your left breast is larger than your right breast.

- Your hair turns reddish.

- Your bump is high up.

- You crave sweets, fruit and orange juice.

- You have mood swings.

- Add your age at the time of conception to the number of the month you conceived. If the amount is odd, it's a girl.

Pocket fact 🔡

Baby boys slightly outnumber baby girls (by about 106 to 100).

A low-lying placenta

*Sometimes the placenta – the amazing organ that acts as a life support system to your baby by passing on oxygen and blood from you – implants low in the uterus and ends up covering, or at least threatening to cover, the cervix (the entrance to the womb). Usually, a low-lying placenta will move out of the way later on in pregnancy, in plenty of time for your baby to be born. But in about 10% of cases, it won't and this is known as a **placenta praevia**. This is a potentially risky condition and your medical team will want to keep a close eye on you. If it's largely, or completely, blocking your baby's exit route, you will almost certainly need to have your baby by **planned Caesarean section** (see pp. 120–21).*

🛒 TESTING FOR DOWN'S 🛒

These days, all pregnant women are offered some form of testing for **Down's syndrome**.

Testing for Down's is completely optional. If tests establish that you *do* have a baby with Down's, you'll have time to weigh up your options – or even just to prepare for the emotional and practical needs of a child with this condition.

Pocket fact 🎲

Your risk of having a baby with Down's increases as you get older – from approximately one in 1,500 for women of 20, to one in 900 for women of 30, to one in 100 for women of 40.

- Screening to show the risk of Down's syndrome is done by blood test, or by ultrasound, or by a combination of both.

- The test will indicate whether you're at high risk or not – only around 3% of tests will throw up this result and it *doesn't* mean for certain that your baby has Down's Syndrome.

- If you do get a high-risk result from this initial screening, you'll be offered a diagnostic test, which will give a more definitive answer but carries with it a slight risk of miscarriage.

- You should get lots of support and information from your midwife or doctor, as this decision can be a tricky one. In the end it's a personal decision and one that only you, and your partner, can make.

- In the majority of cases, the test will be negative. But if the result is a positive one, you should be offered all the advice and support you need to decide what happens next.

Down's syndrome

- *Named after John Langdon Down, the doctor who first identified it, Down's syndrome is a genetic disorder that affects around 1 in 1,000 babies.*
- *A baby born with Down's is likely to have a low birth weight and a number of typical features that include slanting eyes and a flat back to the head. Physical symptoms include floppy joints and poor muscle tone.*
- *Children with Down's usually develop at a slower pace than is normal and will have some degree of learning difficulties.*
- *There's no cure for Down's syndrome, but lots of support and treatment is available that can improve health and quality of life.*
- *Contact details for the Down's Syndrome Association can be found on its website, www.downs-syndrome.org.uk*

Pocket tip

The majority of tests taken during pregnancy reveal all is well. But if a scan finds a significant problem or potential problem, contact ARC, Antenatal Results and Choices, which exists specifically to help people (www.arc-uk.org).

4

YOUR BABY: WEEK BY WEEK

🚼 THE SCIENCE PART 🚼

- Your egg, released during ovulation, and his sperm fuse together to become one cell (known by the term zygote).

- This then divides to form a cluster of cells, which travels down the Fallopian tube to your uterus (womb).

- Two or three days later, implantation occurs – in other words, the fertilised egg settles down into your womb's lining.

- At this point it becomes an embryo, and technically speaking, you're pregnant – but it will be another fortnight before you're likely to suspect it, or can take a test that will let you know for sure.

Pocket fact 🎲

Forget one in a million – your baby's one in 2 million. Up to 2 million sperm can be released and only one is needed to fertilise an egg.

Here's a rough guide to what's going on inside you during those nine magical months. From here on in, we'll be talking in weeks, and so will you, so you better get used to it!

Pocket tip 🗳

Don't forget, pregnancy is officially dated from the first day of your last period — in other words, two weeks prior to conception. So by week six, for example, the life inside you is actually only four weeks old.

🛒 FIRST TRIMESTER 🛒

AT SIX WEEKS

- The tiny embryo in your uterus, safely encased in the amniotic sac, is just 4–6mm – the size of a pea.

- His neural tube – which will eventually become the brain and spine – has already started to develop, his vital organs are in place and his heart has begun to beat.

- He has little 'buds' where his limbs will soon be emerging, an emerging head and dimples that will become his ears.

Pocket fact 🎲

By three weeks after conception, your embryo's heart begins to beat. It's only the size of a poppy seed.

It beats twice as fast as yours throughout your pregnancy, and reaches top speeds of 157 beats per minute at the end of your first trimester.

The placenta

Part of the cluster of cells that implanted will now develop into the placenta (afterbirth) — the organ which links your blood supply to the baby's, and through which oxygen and nutrients are passed from you to your baby via the umbilical cord. The same system carries waste from the baby out again. The placenta also helps protect your baby from infection as it passes on antibodies from you, and produces hormones that will sustain his growth and development in the womb.

The placenta pumps around 35% of the blood in your body to your baby (that's 500ml a minute).

AT EIGHT WEEKS

- Your baby is now a prawn-shaped foetus and is around 1–2cm long.

- Although he's bobbing around in amniotic fluid – a colourless liquid that's helping to protect him in the womb – you won't feel his movements for a while yet, although they could be detected from now by ultrasound scan.

- His face is slowly forming, too, and has small dark splodges where his eyes will be. His skin is transparent and paper-thin.

Pocket fact

The percentage of saline content in amniotic fluid is the same as that of the sea.

AT 10 WEEKS

- Your baby is now around 2–4cm long (this is known as his crown to rump length – in other words, what he measures from head to bottom).

- He has a disproportionately large head, but his body is beginning to straighten.

- His facial features – including the beginnings of nose and upper lip – and limbs continue to grow.

Pocket fact 🎲

Foetus means 'young one'.

AT 12 WEEKS

- He's now fully formed. His skeleton is complete and all his body parts and organs are in place, including the sex organs.

- He can suck, swallow and yawn.

- He continues to be active, but you still won't feel it yet.

- His fingers and toes have separated and his hair is growing – though the colour of it could well change after he's born.

- His eyes are fully formed, but still closed, and his sense of hearing is developing.

- He already has the beginnings of his teeth – even though they won't usually appear until he's five or six months old.

Week 13 is a real turning point in pregnancy: you're through the risky first trimester, when most miscarriages occur, and your chances of losing the baby become very small. It's usual to have a dating scan around now.

🍼 SECOND TRIMESTER 🍼

AT 14 WEEKS

- You're in the second trimester now and your baby's length is approximately 8–10cm.

- He has a recognisable chin, forehead and nose.

- He'll start to develop a fine covering of downy body hair, known as lanugo – there to keep him warm until he's laid down sufficient body fat to do so.

- He has a unique set of fingerprints.

From now, your midwife may use a Doppler – a handheld ultrasound machine – to locate and listen to your baby's heartbeat. A normal foetal heart rate (FHR) can be anywhere between 110 beats and 160 beats per minute, but on average it will be around 140 beats to 150 beats per minute – twice as fast as a normal adult's.

Pocket fact 🎲
On average a baby will go through 7,500 nappies in a year.

AT 16 WEEKS

- He can wave his fingers, toes and limbs around now.

- He has little fingernails in place and he may be able to suck his thumb.

- His ears are developing and he can hear your voice, as well as your heartbeat and the rumblings and grumblings of your digestive system.

You may just about be able to make out your baby's movement from now onwards. At first it feels rather like a fluttering or bubbling sensation, very easily confused with indigestion. Don't worry if you can't feel anything yet – it's still early days, and you should pick up on them some time in the next four to six weeks.

AT 18 WEEKS

- He's 13cm to 15cm in length now.

- He can punch, kick, turn and wriggle.

- His head is still large in comparison with his body, but his face is becoming more and more human in appearance. He's also pulling a range of faces.

- Although his eyes are still shut, they'll be sensitive to bright lights from outside.

- He's begun to practise his breathing skills in preparation for his exit, by inhaling and exhaling amniotic fluid.

Pocket fact 🏠

Babies play with their umbilical cord. Research suggests they give themselves what's thought to be an early adrenaline buzz by grasping it hard enough to cause a brief restriction to their oxygen supply.

AT 20 WEEKS

- He's beginning to get a waxy coating known as 'vernix' to protect his skin from the soaking it's getting – most will be gone by the time he's born, but there may well be traces left.

- His hearing is well developed and he may jump or jerk at loud noises.

- His taste buds are developing.

- He'll be growing eyelashes and eyebrows.

Pocket fact

Now your baby's passing about 3tbsp of urine a day made up of the amniotic fluid he swallows, which is about 2 litres a day!

You're halfway there and you should be offered an anomaly scan now or very soon. It's usually possible for the sonographer to tell the sex of your baby (fairly accurately – but it's not guaranteed). However, you might have to ask for this information – and some hospitals still have a policy of not letting on at all.

AT 22 WEEKS

- Your baby's crown to rump measurement will be somewhere around 18cm to 20cm now.

- His head and body size have evened out so he's in proportion.

- He can hear noises outside the womb and will hear mother's voice clearer than anything, so start talking or singing to him.

Pocket fact

One in every 2,000 babies is born with a tooth.

AT 24 WEEKS

- His lungs are strengthening and he'll be practising his breathing by inhaling and exhaling amniotic fluid (sometimes causing him to have hiccups, which you can feel!).

- His skin will still be wrinkly, as he's yet to plump out to his full weight.

- He has fully formed eyes.

From this week, your baby is considered to be viable, which means if born, he'd stand a chance of survival with intensive care in a neonatal unit.

AT 26 WEEKS

- He'll open his eyes for the first time around now.

- You'll probably be well aware of all his somersaults, kicks and karate chops.

🛒 THIRD TRIMESTER 🛒

Pocket fact 🎲
Your baby will now put on half a pound a day.

AT 28 WEEKS

- His brain continues to develop and it's thought that babies may begin to dream around now.

- Visual responses are up and running – if you were to shine a torch at your belly, he'd turn his head to find out who put the lights on.

- His transparent skin is beginning to turn opaque.

AT 30 WEEKS

- Your baby should now be around 28cm long and weighing an average of 3lbs.

- His wrinkly skin will be smoothing out as he gets plumper.

- His lungs and digestive tract are almost fully formed.

Pocket fact 🎲

At this point, your baby can tell light from dark. So, if you move a torch across your stomach, your baby will notice.

Your baby's movement

You may find your baby becomes less active than he has been. It's nothing to worry about; it's just because there's less room in there. It's very normal for movement to be erratic and you probably won't need to panic.

The general guideline given is that you should feel 10 or more kicks in a day, but more important than that is getting to know your baby's own pattern, so you notice if it changes.

If you haven't felt a normal amount of movement from your baby during his usually most active period, sit quietly and drink a glass of iced water – as your bladder fills up, it should provoke some movement. If it doesn't, and you're still concerned, let your midwife know.

AT 32 WEEKS

- He may be lying head down in preparation for birth by now, but there's still loads of time for him to turn.

- His sleeping cycles may be longer, so you may notice he's quieter for longer periods.

- The lanugo (hair) covering his body will now begin to fall out.

Your midwife will be keeping an eye on your baby's position by feeling your abdomen carefully during your routine checks: if your baby doesn't get into the right position as you get closer to your EDD, your obstetrician may carry out a procedure called an external cephalic version (ECV) to avoid a breech birth (see p. 121).

> *Pocket fact* 🎲
>
> *The average gestation period is 266 days.*

AT 34 WEEKS

- Your baby now measures somewhere around 32cm in length and weighs about 5lbs.

- He can open and close his eyes and focus on his own fingers in front of him.

- Most of his organs are now fully mature, except for his lungs.

- He's built up some fat deposits under his skin, making it appear pink rather than red.

There's not a lot of room left in your uterus now and you may be getting prodded and poked to a quite uncomfortable extent. You can also try to feel or see an elbow or foot protruding from down below, or watch as his movements cause ripples across the surface of your tummy.

AT 36 WEEKS

- His brain and nervous system are now fully developed and his bones are beginning to harden – although the skull remains soft and flexible (hence the soft spot that your baby will have for up to 18 months after his birth) so that he can make it through the birth canal.

- If your baby is a boy, his testicles will normally have begun their descent from the abdomen into the scrotum.

- His lungs are now almost fully developed and in a week's time he'll be officially full-term. If born, he'd almost certainly survive without major problems and may not even need any special care.

Most babies will have moved into the 'head-first' position by now but a small number remain in the 'breech' (bottom first) position, or even sideways (transverse). You may soon feel pressure low in your abdomen, caused by the 'engagement' process, as the baby drops down in preparation for birth. Some babies don't engage until the last minute, though.

Pocket fact 🔡

Babies born with their amniotic sac intact are said to be 'born in the caul' and are believed to be lucky.

AT 38 WEEKS

- He's likely to be around 6lbs to 7lbs in weight now and is definitely full-term (some experts classify 37 weeks as full-term, others 38).

- He'll have lost most or all of his hairy, waxy coatings (actually, he has swallowed them and will poo them out after he's born.)

- He won't be moving so vigorously, he just doesn't have room!

It's time to be on your guard for signs of labour – see p. 145.

AT 40 WEEKS

- He's an average 35cm to 37cm from crown to rump.
- He weighs anything from 6lbs to 8lbs on average.
- He's got fully developed internal organs.
- If you haven't yet gone into labour, you soon will!

Pocket fact 🎲

Your uterus is now 500–1,000 times its normal size!
*   It started off the size of a small Conference pear; now it's more like an oversized watermelon.*

Some pregnancies go on for 42 weeks or even 43 weeks. Your midwife will be keeping a very close eye from now on – sometimes when a baby's deliberating his arrival, labour may need a helping hand (see pp. 143–44).

🛒 TWINS OR MULTIPLES 🛒

FINDING OUT IT'S TWINS

Pocket fact 🎲

In the UK about one in 80 babies is born a twin or triplet.

- It is possible for the sonographer to see if you are carrying twins at your dating scan, although it is possible for this to be missed. It depends what position the babies are lying in.
- The sonographer will look for two heartbeats (not including yours) and also extra limbs.

- They will look for two amniotic sacs, which are both growing at around the same speed.

Pocket fact 🎲

One in four births from IVF conceptions results in twins or multiples.

WHAT WILL IT CHANGE?

You might be very surprised and worry that you won't be able to cope with two (or more) babies. This is a natural reaction and, just like when you found out you were pregnant, the news can take time to sink in.

Pocket fact 🎲

Between 1996 and 2006 there was a 182% increase of twins in pregnancies when the mother was over 35.

Your pregnancy will be affected by this news:

- You'll probably be bigger than women carrying just one baby (even though twins are smaller).

- You'll be more tired.

- You might suffer from morning sickness and other pregnancy ailments more.

- You'll have to eat more (roughly 600 calories more than usual a day, as opposed to a normal pregnancy's 200–300 more calories).

Pocket fact 🧱
The most babies born in a single birth is nine.

Carrying more than one baby around will mean a few things practically too:

- Twins have a habit of coming early, so make sure you're prepared for the birth and have your hospital bag packed by week 32 – just in case. Think about starting your maternity leave a bit early.

Pocket fact 🧱
22% of twins are left-handed compared to about 10% of non-twins.

- Consider what support you'll need. Do you need to enlist a family member to help you in the first few weeks? Or hire in some help? Join an online community to allay your fears.

- Reassess your finances – don't assume you have to buy two of everything, but consider what will change with two mouths to feed.

Pocket tip 🤚
If you're pregnant through IVF, you will have a scan four or five weeks into your pregnancy. Your chances of having multiples are 20 times higher than a natural conception. Twenty-four per cent of IVF babies are multiples.

5

YOUR BODY: GOING THROUGH CHANGES

You'll experience a number of changes to your body during your pregnancy.

- As a very general rule, you can expect most of the worst symptoms to strike during the first trimester, when the pregnancy hormones are at their most active.

- The second trimester is usually considered the best, health wise, where you 'bloom' because you're no longer plagued by the hormones.

- During the third trimester, the biggest challenge will be your ever increasing bump.

We've listed the body changes in alphabetical order for ease of finding them, and given you practical advice on how you can relieve each ailment.

Pocket tip ☞
If you're in any doubt at all, ask your midwife, or make an appointment with your GP. Remember it's their job to help you, so don't feel embarrassed about anything.

If you need an answer quickly, try 24-hour NHS Direct: 0845 46 47.

There are some symptoms that you should seek advice on urgently, listed on p. 61.

🍼 ABDOMINAL PAIN 🍼

It's not unusual to feel pains in your stomach during pregnancy that don't signal a major problem. Early on, there can be a little period-like pain as the embryo implants in your womb. It can also be caused by the uterus growing and stretching and, later, simply by the pressure caused by your growing baby. A sharp, stabbing pain in the side or groin is common in the last trimester, caused by the stretching of the muscles and ligaments around the uterus. This may also be **constipation** or **wind** (see below).

What can I do about it?

Not very much. Sit down and get some rest.

Could it be serious?

Generally, tummy pains are only cause for concern if they are very severe, and/or you have some other symptom alongside it, such as regular, rhythmic tightening of your abdomen, bleeding, a high temperature, chills, vomiting, blood in the urine or pain urinating.

Pocket fact 🔡

The hormone progesterone increases during pregnancy.

🍼 ANAEMIA 🍼

In most cases, anaemia during pregnancy is caused by iron deficiency. This can lead to symptoms such as exhaustion, palpitations, headaches, dizziness and shortness of breath. It can also make you more prone to infections.

What can I do about it?

Make sure you eat plenty of foods that are rich in iron (see p. 86). Your GP or midwife could give you iron tablets.

Could it be serious?

In most cases anaemia won't be a major problem. However, severe anaemia may increase the risk of a postpartum haemorrhage.

Pocket fact 🔠

Back pain is really common during pregnancy, affecting as many as three-quarters of women.

🍼 BACK PAIN 🍼

Pregnant bodies release a hormone called relaxin, with the aim of making the joints and ligaments – especially in the pelvic region – more flexible in preparation for birth. This can make the lower back painful. And it's not helped by your baby's weight.

What can I do about it?

- Regular, gentle exercise such as yoga, pilates or swimming.

- Strengthen your abdominal muscles, as they perform such an important role in supporting your back: try doing some pelvic tilts (see p. 92).

- Pay attention to your posture: try to avoid standing for long periods and avoid lifting anything heavy. Check the position of your computer and chair if you work at a desk.

- Try a maternity support belt, band or corset – these are made from stretchy fabric and have a wider panel that sits underneath the bump to give it support.

- Massage can help, although it's generally recommended that you avoid it in the first trimester.

- If it's very bad, your doctor may prescribe pain relief medication or refer you to a physiotherapist or other specialist.

Could it be serious?

For some women, back pain in pregnancy can be very severe. Let your midwife know if you're really suffering – sooner rather than later.

🚼 BLEEDING GUMS 🚼

Changing hormone levels cause the gums to swell and become more sensitive than usual and, in some cases, this can lead to soreness and bleeding – known as gingivitis.

What can I do about it?

Brush your teeth and gums twice daily with a fluoride toothpaste for at least two minutes, and floss (even if to do so makes them bleed more).

Could it be serious?

If left untreated, gingivitis can cause major decay to teeth and gums.

Pocket tip 🖘
Don't forget that NHS dental care is free when you're pregnant, so make the most of it. Get the exemption form from your midwife.

🍼 BIGGER, TENDER BREASTS 🍼

Changing hormones, increasing blood flow and the beginnings of milk production all contribute to bigger, and often painful, breasts in the first trimester.

What can I do about it?

Get yourself fitted for a new, comfortable, practical bra – chances are you've gone up by at least a cup size. If you're in a lot of discomfort, wear a soft cotton sleep bra at night, too.

A little gentle massage can ease tenderness – if you can bear to be touched.

Could it be serious?

Only for your other half if he tries to cop a feel when they're sore!

Pocket tip 🍵

You should aim to be measured several times during pregnancy, as your assets may swell by up to three cup sizes overall.

🍼 BREATHLESSNESS 🍼

Breathlessness *is* very normal, and occurs because your lungs are having to work harder to provide extra oxygen – and also when, later in pregnancy, your growing uterus pushes against your diaphragm.

What can I do about it?

Not a lot. It's normal and harmless, but if an attack of breathlessness occurs, don't panic; sit down and rest.

Could it be serious?

No, but do let your midwife know if you're experiencing it with any other symptoms alongside, such as palpitations or chest pain.

👶 CONSTIPATION 👶

This is common for two reasons during pregnancy: hormones relax the digestive system, which slows down the movement of food through it, and your growing uterus puts pressure on your bowels.

What can I do about it?

- Eat plenty of fibre-rich foods such as wholemeal bread, fruit and vegetables and pulses.

- Drink lots of water.

- Regular gentle exercise like walking and swimming will help.

- If it is really bad, a gentle laxative treatment may help, but be sure to get a prescription from your doctor or midwife as some laxatives are too strong for safe use in pregnancy.

Could it be serious?

No, although it can be very uncomfortable.

👶 CRAMPS 👶

Sudden spasms of pains in the legs and feet. It's not clear why these happen, but theories include muscle fatigue; a deficiency of minerals; and pressure on the nerves caused by the growing uterus.

What can I do about it?

Try not to cross your legs when sitting or standing. Keep your legs and ankles moving by stretching and wiggling your calves and feet. If you do get cramp, stretch out the leg and rotate your ankle, or try walking around the room. Gently rub the muscle. Eat a balanced diet – this may help boost any minerals you're missing.

Could it be serious?

No, they'll only come in short, temporary bursts and won't last beyond pregnancy. If you've got severe, persistent leg pain and/or you're suffering from other symptoms such as swelling of the leg, contact your GP as this could be a sign of a **deep vein thrombosis** (see below).

🛒 DEEP VEIN THROMBOSIS 🛒

On average, one in every 1,000 women will get a venous thrombosis (a blood clot in the vein) during pregnancy or just after birth.

Deep vein thrombosis (DVT) is when a blood clot occurs in a deep vein, usually in the leg, and this is the most common sort of clot to affect pregnant women.

Symptoms of deep vein thrombosis include pain, tenderness and swelling in the leg, which may turn pale blue or reddish purple in colour. If you notice any of these, do alert your midwife or doctor immediately.

You can get more information from Lifeblood, the thrombosis charity: www.thrombosis-charity.org.uk

Pocket fact 🔲

In the last trimester you could be lugging around the equivalent of up to seven bags of sugar (taking into account the weight of baby, uterus, placenta and amniotic fluid).

🚼 EXHAUSTION 🚼

It's common to feel exhausted in the first trimester and, later on, as you carry around all that extra weight. It's made worse when combined with other common features of pregnancy such as **insomnia**, **nausea**, poor diet, or a lack of exercise.

What can I do about it?

Not much, other than resting, getting early nights and delegating tiring matters such as housework.

Could it be serious?

No.

🚼 FAINTING OR DIZZINESS 🚼

Your body's increased demand for blood and, later on, the pressure of the growing womb on the blood vessels can cause dizzy spells and faintness. Other factors linked to pregnancy such as tiredness, dehydration, overheating, and low blood sugar can also contribute.

What can I do about it?

Keep a snack on you at all times when you're out and about to give your blood sugar levels a boost if necessary. If you feel faint, lie down with your feet up, or sit with your head in between your knees. Wear layers so you can avoid getting too hot, which can trigger fainting.

Could it be serious?

If it's happening a lot, you might have **anaemia**, and it's also a symptom of **gestational diabetes**. Do mention it to your midwife.

🚼 FORGETFULNESS, OR 🚼 'BABY BRAIN'

Anecdotal evidence suggests as many as half of pregnant women suffer from 'baby brain' (also known as 'preg-head') during pregnancy, but little reliable scientific research has been carried out on the subject.

What can I do about it?

Nothing – other than writing yourself lots of lists.

Could it be serious?

No.

🚼 HAIRINESS 🚼

You may find that you have increased hair growth during pregnancy, over your whole body. However, some women find it works the other way and they have less body hair, or that some of the hair on their head falls out.

What can I do about it?

- Waxing, plucking and shaving are all fine, but do a patch test before using a hair removal cream as skin tends to be more sensitive during pregnancy.

- Although there's no evidence that electrolysis and laser treatment can be harmful to a baby, some practitioners advise against it.

- You might find you're better off relaxing about hairier body parts.

Could it be serious?

No.

Pocket fact 🎲

There's no truth in the pregnancy myth that a hairy belly means you're having a boy . . .

🍼 HEADACHES 🍼

Frequent headaches during pregnancy are common, but their cause isn't really understood. Hormones and the change in blood supply are probable culprits and other factors like **nausea** and dehydration, **nasal congestion**, **insomnia** and stress may also play a part.

What can I do about it?

- Try to find a moment to lie down, preferably in the dark, and rest.

- Doctors generally advise against any sort of medication in pregnancy, and aspirin and ibuprofen are out, but moderate doses of paracetamol are okay.

- Aim for prevention rather than cure by getting as much sleep and rest as possible, eating well and drinking plenty of fluids. Avoid caffeine.

Could it be serious?

If you're getting severe headaches or migraines, or you're having other symptoms alongside such as blurred vision, vomiting or swelling, do mention it to your midwife as there's a chance the symptoms could indicate **pre-eclampsia**.

Pre-eclampsia

Raised blood pressure is very common in pregnancy, but up to 1 in 10 women will develop pre-eclampsia, a potentially serious form of pregnancy-related high blood pressure. You're more likely to get it if:

- *it's your first pregnancy*
- *you are over 40*
- *you are obese*
- *you have a family history of it*
- *you have suffered from high blood pressure before becoming pregnant anyway*
- *you are having twins.*

It will only develop after 20 weeks and is likely to be detected during routine antenatal tests on your blood pressure and urine.

You'll be closely monitored if you're found to have high blood pressure at any stage. You'll be advised to eat healthily and stay active, and you may be offered medication that can reduce your blood pressure.

Symptoms of pre-eclampsia may include headaches, swelling in the hands and feet, blurred vision and vomiting.

For more detailed information, visit the website of Action on Pre-eclampsia (www.apec.org.uk).

🚼 INCONTINENCE 🚼

Inevitably, the pelvic floor muscle – which supports the bladder – comes under a lot of stress during pregnancy as the uterus grows. Leaking urine when you cough, laugh, sneeze or jump up and down is a problem that affects many.

What can I do about it?

Regular pelvic floor exercises (see p. 93). Don't be tempted to cut out fluids, as it's important to keep well hydrated for good health.

Could it be serious?

It should get better after pregnancy – but birth itself can damage the pelvic floor further. All of which emphasises the importance of pelvic floor exercises.

🚼 INDIGESTION AND HEARTBURN 🚼

Indigestion – pain or discomfort in the chest and upper tummy – and heartburn – a burning pain in the stomach, chest and throat – are extremely common during pregnancy and they occur for two reasons: hormones cause the digestive system to relax, which leads to excess acid into the stomach; and, later on, the growing womb is putting pressure on the stomach.

What can I do about it?

- Try eating smaller meals and eating slowly.

- Cut out whichever foods are most to blame: spicy, fatty and processed foods are usual.

- At night, try sleeping in a propped-up position using pillows.

- Some women report that drinking milk can help reduce the acid.

- Also try a suitable over-the-counter antacid remedy such as Gaviscon – ask your midwife to recommend one.

Could it be serious?

No, just uncomfortable.

Pocket fact

If you have indigestion, it doesn't mean you're going to have a hairy baby!

INSOMNIA

Likely culprits for insomnia are: back pain, overactive bladders, heartburn, and your growing belly, which makes it hard to find a comfy position. As many pregnant women are anxious, they find they have strange dreams and are wide awake worrying.

What can I do about it?

Make yourself as comfortable as possible – a pillow between the legs and one under your bump can really help. Avoid caffeine at night. Try to get a little exercise in the evening, or at least try some relaxation and breathing techniques (see p. 92).

ITCHING

Mild itching is normal and is caused because of the increased blood flow to the skin, also, later on, as the skin stretches across your growing belly. Pregnancy hormones also make the skin more sensitive than usual and therefore more prone to rashes and itchy patches.

What can I do about it?

Wear loose clothing made of natural fibres and try using a gentle, soothing cream such as calamine lotion.

Could it be serious?

Severe itching, particularly in unusual places such as the palms of hands or soles of feet, can *occasionally* indicate a potentially serious liver condition called **obstetric cholestasis** (see below), so keep your midwife informed.

Obstetric cholestasis

Obstetric cholestasis is a liver disorder that causes a leakage of bile into the bloodstream. The causes are unknown, although it's believed to run in families.

It's thought to affect 1 in 160 pregnant women, and is more common with multiples.

The most common symptom, which usually doesn't develop until the third trimester, is itching, often worst on the hands and feet. But it can also cause tiredness, mild jaundice, dark urine and a lack of appetite. Because studies in the past have linked the condition with an increased risk of stillbirth, women who are diagnosed are closely monitored and usually offered an induction at 37 weeks or 38 weeks.

Obstetric cholestasis is purely pregnancy-related and will cease to be a problem once your baby is born. Visit the Obstetric Cholestasis Support website (www.ocsupport.org.uk) for more information.

MOOD SWINGS

It's totally normal to feel miserable as your hormones take their toll emotionally as well as physically. Naturally, you may be worried or anxious about many things. And if you're suffering from any other physical symptoms that'll affect your mood.

What can I do about it?

Keep your chin up: mood swings are common in the first trimester but will usually subside. Try to get as much rest and sleep as you can. Look for distractions: a good book or movie, some relaxation exercises (see p. 92).

Could it be serious?

A certain amount of mood swinging is very normal, but it's known that women who feel very down during pregnancy are at higher risk of developing postnatal depression after the birth, so do mention it to your GP.

'MORNING' SICKNESS OR NAUSEA

> *Pocket fact*
>
> *Morning sickness is experienced by as many as 85% of pregnant women.*

'Morning' sickness is a total misnomer, since it very often lasts all day. For some women it involves actual vomiting, whilst for others it goes no further than the distinct feeling that they're about to. It can be one of the worse elements of early pregnancy.

Appetite is often affected; in fact, some women find they can't face food at all – and then worry about the lack of nutrition they, and their baby, are getting. It usually (although not always) eases up once the first trimester is over.

What can I do about it?

- Do try to keep eating if you can – little and often, if you can't face full meals.

- Experiment to try to find things that you can stomach – anything spicy or greasy is probably best avoided.

- If you can't eat at all, remember to drink instead to avoid dehydration – especially if you are actually vomiting.

- Ginger is an alternative remedy that is believed to help – try nibbling ginger biscuits, or drinking hot water infused with real ginger root.

- You could try an acupressure band, which is worn around the wrist and is said to relieve nausea by pushing down on a particular pressure point. They're available from larger chemists and health food shops.

Could it be serious?

Morning sickness won't harm your baby, who'll still thrive, even if you've eaten nothing but ginger nuts and mashed potato for three months. Excessive vomiting can lead to severe dehydration and need hospital treatment, so talk to your GP or midwife if it gets really bad. Also seek help if you have vomiting that's accompanied by other symptoms, such as fever or pain, in case it's being caused by a completely different medical problem.

Pocket fact 🔡

Morning sickness is believed to indicate high levels of the hormone human chorionic gonadotrophin (hCG) — this is the stuff that's nourishing your baby until the placenta takes over the job at around 12 weeks. There's a theory that morning sickness gives you a lower risk of miscarriage. (Please note, though, this is no reason to fret if you aren't experiencing morning sickness — not all women do.)

👶 NOSE BLEEDS AND 👶 NASAL CONGESTION

The increased blood supply of pregnancy puts pressure on the veins inside the nose and causes the sinuses to swell, which makes them more prone to bleeding and/or nasal congestion (as well as snoring).

What can I do about it?

- Remain upright and pinch your nose gently but firmly for up to 10 minutes, which should stop the flow — if not, repeat.

- Take care to blow your nose gently when you need to.

- Stuffiness can be relieved with a little steam inhalation — put a kettle full of hot water in the sink, cover your head with a towel and take a few deep breaths.

- If it gets bad, your doctor may prescribe a safe decongestant.

Could it be serious?

It's likely to be a harmless annoyance. But frequent or heavy nose-bleeds can be a sign of **anaemia**, so if they're bad, seek help.

🛒 PAIN IN THE HANDS 🛒

Lots of pregnant women experience this, medical term carpal tunnel syndrome (CTS). It's caused by a build-up of fluid in the tube that houses the wrist nerves and leads to pain, throbbing, numbness or pins and needles in the hands and fingers. It commonly gets worse at night.

What can I do about it?

Rest and raise the hands as much as possible. If you're really suffering, you should be referred to a physiotherapist.

Could it be serious?

In most cases it eases after the baby is born.

🛒 PELVIC PAIN 🛒

The pelvic joints loosen in pregnancy to allow room for the baby's exit. This causes discomfort and/or pain in the pelvic region as well as in the buttocks, hips, legs and lower back for many women. There may also be an audible clicking or grinding sound when you move. This condition is widely known now as pregnancy-related pelvic girdle pain, or PGP. It can strike at any point in pregnancy and sometimes just afterwards.

What can I do about it?

- Rest – try to lie down whenever you can – and avoid activities that lead to pain.

- Pay attention to your posture: aim to keep your knees close together and when standing, try to keep straight so your weight is evenly distributed over both legs.

- If PGP is causing significant discomfort or pain, your doctor may prescribe painkillers or refer you to a physiotherapist, who will suggest exercises that can help and can provide equipment such as a pelvic support belt, or crutches, if necessary.

- Some women report that alternative treatments such as cranial osteopathy provide considerable relief.

Could it be serious?

For some women, PGP can become so severe it makes ordinary activities such as walking, making love and even turning over in bed agony. It also has implications for the birth and for caring for your baby afterwards, since the symptoms can continue after pregnancy. In these cases a referral for physiotherapy will be vital.

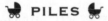 PILES

Piles (officially known as haemorrhoids) are a common irritant of pregnancy. These little lumpy clusters around the back passage are caused when the veins there swell and the result may be pain or itching. They may also bleed and usually cause pain or discomfort when you're trying to do a poo (which can exacerbate the problem and cause a vicious circle if you're already suffering from **constipation**).

What can I do about it?

Eat lots of fibre and drink plenty of water to keep your bowel movements loose and regular. An ice pack or cold flannel can provide a little relief. You could also ask your midwife or doctor to recommend a suitable over-the-counter cream or, if they're severe, to prescribe suppositories.

Could it be serious?

No.

🍼 RESTLESS LEG SYNDROME 🍼

Restless leg syndrome (RLS) can affect anyone at any time, but doctors are unclear why it's more common during pregnancy. It's an uncomfortable, sometimes painful, urge to move the legs and a feeling that your legs are 'tingling', 'crawling' or 'burning'. It usually strikes when you're resting, especially at the end of the day. Symptoms are usually eased by moving or massaging the legs but return again when you're resting – so it can make it hard to get to sleep.

What can I do about it?
Try cutting out alcohol and caffeine entirely and aim to relax in the evenings.

Could it be serious?
No.

🍼 RIB PAIN 🍼

Sore and tender ribs can occur, generally later on in the third trimester, as your uterus expands and pushes against the ribs. The baby can also cause a fair amount of pain with kicking, punching and head-butting.

What can I do about it?
Stick to loose clothing and keep an eye on your posture. A mound of well-placed cushions can aid your comfort while sitting.

Could it be serious?
No.

Pocket fact 🔡

Babies born to women over the age of 40 are 28% more likely to be left-handed.

🍼 SKIN CHANGES 🍼

All sorts of odd things can happen to your skin because of hormonal changes.

- Changes in pigmentation can cause dark patches on the face – or, if you're dark skinned, lighter patches – sometimes called 'the mask of pregnancy'.

- You may also notice moles, freckles and birthmarks, and your areolae (the skin around the nipple) darkening.

- A dark line running down the centre of your tummy – known as the 'linea nigra' – can appear.

- Increased levels of blood can make your skin appear rosier than usual (hence the 'blooming' during pregnancy) and can also sometimes lead to the appearance of spider veins – small clusters of broken capillaries on the face and body.

- Some women find they get spotty, since hormones drive an increased production of sebum, the oily substance that keeps our skin supple.

What can I do about it?

Not much. Most skin changes don't cause any harm and will fade back to normal after pregnancy. You could cover up patches, spider veins and high colour with a good foundation and tackle oiliness with a really thorough cleansing regime.

Could it be serious?

No.

🛒 SMELL, HEIGHTENED SENSE OF 🛒

Many pregnant women report that their sense of smell becomes very sensitive. It's thought this could be down to the same rush of hormones that (probably) cause morning sickness.

What can I do about it?

Nothing, really.

Could it be serious?

No.

Pocket fact 🔡

It's not uncommon for a woman to dislike the smell of her own partner during pregnancy — no one knows why this is.

🛒 STRETCH MARKS 🛒

Pink or purplish lines appear on the belly, or anywhere else where you gain weight during pregnancy, such as breasts or thighs. They affect some women and not others: it's all down to genetic factors, so if you're going to get them, you're going to get them.

What can I do about them?

Nothing (apart from surgery). There are creams and oils available that claim to help in preventing them, but these aren't proven to work. They usually fade a certain amount over time, but will probably be visible for life – unless you can afford that tummy tuck.

Could it be serious?

No, but it doesn't help your post-baby body esteem.

🚼 SWOLLEN ANKLES, 🚼 FEET AND FINGERS

This is common and is caused by displaced fluids that have been forced elsewhere in the body by the increased blood flow. It can be made worse if the weather's warm or you've been standing for long periods.

What can I do about it?

- Don't stand up for too long – rest and put your feet up whenever you can.

- Try rotating your foot regularly, to both sides.

- A good pair of support tights can also minimise the risks.

Could it be serious?

Generally this is harmless. But do keep an eye on it and mention it to your midwife, as severe swelling in the hands and face can be a symptom of **pre-eclampsia** (see p. 44).

🚼 THRUSH 🚼

During pregnancy, the natural balance of bacteria in the vagina is affected by hormones, which means you're up to 10 times more likely to get thrush.

What can I do about it?

- Eating natural yoghurt is said to keep thrush at bay because it contains infection-busting organisms – you can also apply it directly on your bits for some soothing (but very messy) relief.

- Antifungal creams and pessaries are available on prescription or over the counter – some thrush treatments aren't suitable during pregnancy, though, so check with your doctor or the pharmacist first.

- Avoid wearing tights and tight trousers, and stick to cotton pants. Avoid perfumed shower gels and soaps, which make the irritation worse.

Could it be serious?

No.

Pocket fact 🎲

Actress Kate Winslet confessed that she felt more like a London bus than a film star towards the end of her pregnancy.

🚼 URINATING (LOTS) 🚼

This can kick in early on in pregnancy because of hormone changes and because there's a lot more fluid in the body generally during pregnancy, as the kidneys step up a gear to rid the body of waste products. It usually eases up after the third trimester but often returns with a vengeance later, due to the growing pressure on the bladder caused by your expanding womb.

What can I do about it?

Not much.

- Don't be tempted to hold it in.

- Make sure you've always got access to a loo.

- Empty your bladder comprehensively each time you pee, by 'rocking' backwards and forwards on the toilet a little.

- Don't be tempted to stop drinking, as we all need lots of fluids to keep us healthy – although you could try cutting them down or out late in the evening to avoid a disturbed night.

- Avoid or cut down on anything containing caffeine, as it has a diuretic effect (ie encourages urine flow).

Could it be serious?

Not in itself, but be wary of symptoms such as bloody or cloudy wee, or pain when urinating, which could signal an infection.

VAGINAL DISCHARGE

It's normal to have more vaginal discharge than usual during pregnancy – driven by your hormones, it's nature's way of helping to protect against infections that could travel up to your uterus. It could also be a sign of **cervical erosion** (see **vaginal bleeding**, below). And late in pregnancy you may get a thick 'show' of discharge, which could include some blood and is a sign that labour's imminent (see p. 145).

What can I do about it?

Nothing, there's no need. Avoid washing with perfumed soaps or shower gels and never douche (ie forcefully aim a jet of water up there) as it can upset the balance of chemicals in the vagina and increase your risk of infection. Wear a panty liner (never a tampon).

Could it be serious?

Keep an eye on any heavy discharge – if it becomes dark in colour or smells odd, mention it to your midwife or GP in case you've got some kind of infection, such as **thrush** (see above). A watery discharge in late pregnancy should definitely be reported: it could be leaking amniotic fluid, which could signal **premature rupture of the membranes** (see p. 56).

👶 VARICOSE VEINS 👶

Swollen, bulgy veins that cause pain or itching are a common feature of pregnancy, as the hormones cause the blood vessels to relax and the body's increased blood flow and growing uterus put pressure on the veins. They're most common on the legs, in the anus (where they're better known as **piles**, see above), and inside the vagina. Being overweight and hereditary factors can increase your chance of suffering from them. Women carrying multiples are also more at risk.

What can I do about it?

- Put your feet up – literally. This can help ease the pressure.

- Make sure you get regular rests if you need to stand up for work.

- Support tights or stockings can offer some relief.

- An ice pack (or bag of frozen peas) may prove soothing.

- It's also sensible to exercise gently and keep active to boost your circulation.

Could it be serious?

No, just painful. They'll usually go away or go down at some point after the baby's born.

Pocket fact 🎲

After Sarah Jessica Parker announced she was pregnant the shoe designer Manolo Blahnik designed a new range of kitten heel shows especially for pregnant women.

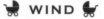 WIND

Hormones play havoc with a pregnant woman's digestive system – compounded later on by the pressure of the growing uterus on the stomach – and, as well as **constipation** and **indigestion**, one of the end results of this is an increase in bloating and wind.

What can I do about it?

Specific foods can make things worse, so you could try pinpointing the usual suspects and removing them from your diet. Eat small meals and take care to chew your food before swallowing. Keeping active can help, too.

Could it be serious?

No.

'My bottom looked like purple sprouting broccoli, other body parts resembled squashes. I was an absolute sight, I really was. How can you feel blooming and sexy when you look like the back end of a bus?!'

Kate Winslet

When to get help – quickly

Some symptoms could (although they won't necessarily) indicate a serious problem and should be checked out as soon as possible. Get on the phone to your midwife or make a same-day appointment with your GP if you're experiencing one or more of the following:

- *Vaginal bleeding (although a little bleeding is not unusual in the early months, and not necessarily a bad sign. See the box below for more on bleeding).*
- *Severe, persistent abdominal pain.*
- *Any kind of vision disturbance.*
- *Sudden or severe swelling in the hands, face and eyes, especially if you also have a headache.*
- *A sudden raging thirst, accompanied by a lack of urination.*
- *Very severe vomiting coupled with pain and/or fever.*
- *Fluid leaking from the vagina.*
- *A severe headache that persists for more than a few hours.*
- *Pain or burning when you wee.*
- *Severe itching all over your body.*
- *A lack of foetal movements after about 20 weeks (see p. 28).*
- *Frequent dizziness or fainting spells.*
- *A heavy fall – although your baby is well cushioned inside you in his amniotic sac, it's best to be checked out after any significant knock.*

If you're very concerned, and you can't get hold of a medical professional, dial 999.

Bleeding in pregnancy

The appearance of any vaginal blood can be a huge worry during pregnancy, but try not to panic if it happens to you – it's common (up to one in five pregnant women experience it) and although you should always take it seriously and get advice, in most cases it will be nothing to worry about. There may not be a cause for bleeding, but where there is, it could be:

- *Implantation bleeding: Some light bleeding, usually known as 'spotting', might appear as the embryo implants in the womb, a few days after conception.*
- *Breakthrough bleeding: Spotting can sometimes occur at around the time your next period – and sometimes subsequent ones – would have been due.*
- *Cervical erosion: The cervix can be affected by cell changes that make it more prone to harmless bleeding (and not because it's 'eroding', in spite of the name). It's also known sometimes as cervical ectropion. If you bleed a little after sex, it will usually be down to this. Cervical erosion may also be the cause of a heavy **vaginal discharge**.*
- *Vaginal infection: **Thrush** (see p. 56), or bacterial vaginosis, can sometimes cause a little bleeding as well as discharge, or a sexually transmitted infection such as chlamydia.*
- *An underlying cause, such as a cervical polyp (a benign growth).*
- ***Placenta praevia:** Where the placenta is low-lying in the uterus and blocks or partially blocks the cervix, from*

where it's more likely to detach and therefore cause bleeding, which may be severe. See p. xx.

- *Placental abruption: A rare complication in which the placenta comes away from its implantation site. It will usually mean an emergency Caesarean section is needed.*
- *Spotting or a bloody 'show' after 37 weeks could just be signs that you're close to going into labour. See p. 62.*
- *Sadly, bleeding does occasionally signal something very serious such as an **ectopic pregnancy**, where the egg has started outside the uterine cavity, most usually in the Fallopian tubes; a **molar pregnancy**, a very rare complication that means the fertilised egg doesn't develop into an embryo, or develops abnormally and can't survive; or a **miscarriage**. Although devastating, miscarriage is common, occurring in up to one in four (recognised) pregnancies, most of those in the first trimester. You can get help and more information from the Miscarriage Association (www.miscarriageassociation.org.uk).*

Do contact your midwife at the first sign of any sort of bleeding.

Pocket fact 🔡
Most women gain between 22lbs and 28lbs during a normal pregnancy.

> **Growing pains**
> *Late pregnancy can be a time of much physical misery. You may well find some of your 'niggles' get even worse — and you may find that you get a whole new set . . .*

🍼 YOUR BUMP 🍼

IS MY BUMP NORMAL?

Bumps can sometimes cause worry, as women fret that theirs is too big, too small, or a strange shape. Remember each bump is unique, and they don't necessarily represent the size and shape of your baby either. What your bump looks like is determined by a range of factors:

- the size of your baby and the placenta
- how much weight you gain
- your height and posture
- the strength of your tummy muscles (the stronger they are the less noticeable your bump will be for a while, and the tighter it will be when it grows — hence in subsequent pregnancies you can generally expect to get bigger, quicker)
- how much amniotic fluid there is
- towards the end — the position of your baby
- if you've got more than one baby in there, that's going to make a difference, too!

Pocket fact 🎲

Demi Moore was photographed naked for the cover of Vanity Fair in August 1991. She is pictured cradling her bump protectively as she turns towards the camera.

WHEN WILL YOU START TO SHOW?

Twelve weeks is probably the earliest you'll 'start to show', as your uterus begins to push out beyond your pubic bone from here on in. Different women will start showing at different times – if you've got a good set of abs on you, or you're very slim, you're more likely to show later than someone who is carrying a bit of extra weight.

Pocket fact 🎲

It's all a myth about the shape and position of your bump being a clue to the gender of your baby. Someone will tell you that if you're carrying it 'all out the front' or 'low-slung', you've got a boy baby in there, whilst 'all round the sides' or 'carrying it high' indicates a girl. Don't believe it.

🍼 FEELING GOOD 🍼

BEAUTY

- **Colouring your hair:** There's no real evidence that colouring your hair will harm your baby – some tests have suggested it may be harmful if absorbed through the scalp and into the bloodstream, but these involved huge quantities of the chemicals in question. So colouring your hair is almost certainly safe.

Pocket tip

It's worth bearing in mind that hormonal changes affect your hair's condition so you might get a different colour or texture from the one you bargained on.

- **Fake tan and sunbeds:** The NHS says it's advisable not to use fake tan during pregnancy because you're more at risk of allergic reactions – you should be fine if you do a patch test first. You're strongly advised not to use a sunbed either.

- **Saunas, hot tubs, steam baths and jacuzzis:** Getting so hot that your body temperature rises isn't recommended. Hot tubs and the like are best avoided, and aim to keep your hot bath water a comfortable temperature.

- **Aromatherapy:** Good for relaxation, but some essential oils are believed to be unsuitable during pregnancy. Use a qualified practitioner who's registered with the Aromatherapy Council.

HOW MUCH WEIGHT SHOULD I GAIN?

It's normal and healthy to gain weight in pregnancy. It varies hugely depending on the size you started out at. The average woman can normally expect to put on anywhere between 22lbs and 28lbs. Only a third of that is accounted for by your baby – the rest is a combination of extra breast tissue, your growing uterus, the placenta, amniotic fluid, increased blood volume, extra fluid and fat stores.

Currently, there aren't any official UK guidelines about what constitutes a healthy weight gain in pregnancy. In the USA, they have a very general rule of thumb based on the 1–2–3 principle:

- If you were overweight before you got pregnant, you should aim to gain no more than a stone.

- If you were a normal weight before you got pregnant, you should aim to gain around 2 stone.

- If you were underweight, you should aim to gain about 3 stone.

> *Pocket fact* 🎲
>
> *The average baby weighs around 7lb 3oz at birth, so by the end of your pregnancy you're carrying half a stone of extra person around with you!*

MATERNITY WEAR

During pregnancy your body will get bigger. That's a given. It's usual for your whole body to get bigger, not just your tummy. This means you'll probably need to rethink your wardrobe. In recent years maternity wear has got much more stylish – but it can be pricey and, since you only need the clothes for a couple of months at a time, not very cost-effective. So you might have to be a bit creative. Here are a few tips:

- Remember to keep anything you buy simple and stylish – that way, if you have another baby, you can reuse the clothes without regretting your purchase.

- Undo the button and zips on your trousers and skirts. You could insert your own stretchy fabric panel (only on clothes you don't want any more). A pair of men's braces can help keep your trousers up if you can't do them up any more.

- Check out charity shops. Look for good-quality maternity wear as well as shirts, tops and skirts in a larger size than you would take normally. If you only fork out a few quid, you can donate them back again once the baby's born and you're (in theory) your old size again.

- Put out a plea on freecycle, a fantastic online community devoted to giving and receiving usable but unwanted stuff (www.freecycle.org). Someone might be looking for a new home for their old maternity wear.

- Borrow stuff from friends who've been pregnant recently. You can always give it back if they want to extend their family later.

- Check out the maternity ranges from cheap and cheerful high street chains like Peacocks and New Look.

- Invest in a couple of good-quality maternity wear basics – most women find at least one pair of pregnancy jeans, which usually come with a stretchy panel, invaluable. (So comfy, in fact, that many choose to hold on to them long after the baby's born.) A pair of black trousers, a smart, forgiving wrap dress and a couple of pretty, empire-line tops are also likely to prove good buys.

- Wear your partner's clothes. But be picky.

- Dress for comfort above all else. Avoid anything with a tight waistband, plump for big, cotton pants, don't dismiss maternity tights and ditch the stilettos.

Pocket fact 🔳

In 2004 a woman in Texas gave birth to two sets of identical twin boys; Jacob and Jacoby, Jason and Justin.

'To be pregnant is to be vitally alive, throughly woman, and undoubtedly inhabited.'

Anne Buchanan

6

LIFESTYLE

🛒 FOOD AND DRINK 🛒

You'll be bombarded with instructions when it comes to your health, and your baby's, and the list of what you should and shouldn't do seems to go on forever. Official guidelines are there with the best of intentions: to warn you of any potential risk (however infinitesimal) that something could pose to baby. But they don't tell you *precisely* what the consequences might be, or how likely they *actually* are. So you end up having to choose between erring comprehensively on the side of caution, or throwing it sometimes to the wind.

So, here's *The Pregnancy Pocket Bible*'s guide to all the official advice on looking after yourself and your baby during pregnancy.

FOOD

There are certain bugs that, if passed on to an unborn baby, could have a harmful effect on them. In pregnancy, your immune system is weakened, which means you're slightly more at risk of picking up infections than usual but, even so, the chances of your baby contracting any of the infections outlined below and being harmed as a result are very small.

Raw or undercooked meat

Undercooked or raw meat can harbour a parasite that can cause an illness called toxoplasmosis. Most of us have already had it and are immune to it, but in a very small number of cases (around 800 babies a year are infected, with 10% of those affected as a result, according to the charity Tommy's), it can lead to serious illness or birth defects in an unborn child, miscarriage or stillbirth.

- Ensure your meat is well cooked, particularly poultry and minced meat products such as sausages and burgers.

- Heat anything that comes from a packet until it's steaming hot all the way through.

- Pay careful attention to food hygiene where raw meat storage and preparation is concerned.

- It's also recommended that you avoid raw meats such as salami, pastrami and parma ham – although these are all fine if cooked, for instance when they're on top of a pizza.

Unwashed fruit, vegetables and salad

Soil on these things may also harbour toxoplasma so official advice is to wash fruit, vegetables and salad well before eating. Wash the packaged, pre-washed varieties just to be on the safe side.

Mould-ripened or blue-veined cheeses

Stilton, Brie, Camembert, Roquefort and Dolcelatte may contain listeria, a bacterium that can cause an infection called listeriosis. It's incredibly rare (infection occurs in one in 30,000 pregnancies, with the chance of harm to your baby even smaller still), and although it may result in nothing more than mild, flu-like symptoms in a pregnant woman, it can lead to serious illnesses such as meningitis, pneumonia or jaundice, premature birth, or even death in an unborn baby.

Raw (unpasteurised) milk or cheeses

These can sometimes harbour bacteria, so you're advised to avoid them in pregnancy. Virtually all the milk and milk products you'll find in the supermarket are pasteurised, and unpasteurised milk is generally only available from specialist suppliers (it's also known as 'green top'), so it's easy enough to avoid. Goat and sheep milk, and their products, are often unpasteurised, so if you rely on it because of an allergy or intolerance to cow's milk, you should double check.

Pregnancy food myth busted

You don't have to give up blue or squidgy cheeses completely if you don't want to. Cooking them through will remove the (already pretty small) risk of listeria, so there's nothing wrong with some deep-fried Brie.

You don't have to avoid all soft cheeses, either, only those that are mould-ripened or made with unpasteurised milk.

Ricotta, mozzarella, mascarpone, cottage cheese, and cream cheese are all absolutely fine.

Raw or undercooked eggs

Undercooked eggs (and poultry) may, just rarely, contain salmonella, leading to food poisoning. It's very unlikely to cause any harm to your baby, but it can also lead to dehydration, which can cause complications.

- Make sure you cook eggs through before consuming. They don't have to be hard boiled – as long as they're lightly cooked, they're fine (see below).

- More of a risk is anything that contains uncooked or partially cooked eggs: homemade versions of mayonnaise, Hollandaise sauce, ice cream, and certain fresh puddings, such as chocolate mousse, for instance – so if you're dining out, you might want to ask first.

- The pre-packaged shop-bought varieties of these things are fine because they'll have been made with pasteurised egg (in other words, heated to a point that would destroy any bacteria).

Pregnancy food myth busted

You don't have to avoid runny or lightly cooked eggs. As long as the whites are no longer translucent, they're cooked enough to be safe. You'll also (almost certainly) be okay if you stick with the 'lion-stamped' eggs as these are inoculated against salmonella. You don't have to avoid mayonnaise, either. As long as it comes out of a jar, it's fine. (And really, does anyone actually make their own?)

Machine ice cream

Soft ice cream that comes out of a machine is best avoided in pregnancy because it's kept at a lower temperature and there's always the risk the machine will be harbouring bacteria. Stick with ice cream from a tub if you want to be certain.

Pocket fact 🎲

In 2004 a set of sextuplets were born in an Ohio hospital in under one minute.

Liver

The official advice is to avoid it altogether as it contains the retinol (animal) form of vitamin A, which can cause birth abnormalities. However, you'd need to eat an awful lot of liver to consume too much retinol, and you've no need to worry if you had some before you knew you were pregnant.

Pregnancy food myth busted

Pro-biotic yoghurts, drinks and other products are all perfectly safe. They do contain bacteria, but only the 'friendly' sort, which are good for us. Sour cream is fine, too.

Shellfish

It's sensible to avoid raw or undercooked shellfish such as prawns, mussels and oysters, as they can harbour bacteria that cause food poisoning such as salmonella. As a general rule, shellfish won't cause you any grief if you cook them before eating, or have them as part of a hot meal, but are probably best avoided from buffets where they may have been hanging around, from fish counters or stalls where you're not sure of the quality, or in ready-prepared sandwiches from sources you don't entirely trust.

Pregnancy food myth busted

You don't have to avoid prawns altogether. They're absolutely fine if heated through (so stir fries and curries are okay). You can also eat them cold as long as they're very fresh, they came pre-packaged and dated (rather than loose), and you eat them the same day.

Raw fish

Advice varies on whether or not you should give up smoked salmon, trout and mackerel during pregnancy. The Food Standards Agency says the risk is negligible, but still stick to the stuff that comes pre-packaged and dated, and refrigerate and eat it quickly.

Sushi gets the go-ahead in general, as it's usually been frozen beforehand, which will kill any parasites that might be hanging around. You'll be okay if you buy it from a supermarket or make it at home (freezing it first, for 24 hours), but if you're in a restaurant, ask first.

Oily fish

Although generally a very nutritious food because it contains omega oils that can help prevent heart disease and may boost the development of an unborn baby's nervous system, don't overdo your consumption of oily fish such as fresh tuna (canned tuna doesn't count as 'oily'), mackerel, salmon, sardines and trout during pregnancy because they've been found to contain pollutants. Food Standards Agency (FSA) guidelines recommend no more than two portions or four cans a week.

Fish with a high mercury content

Fish, such as shark, swordfish or marlin, that may contain mercury, which can damage a baby's nervous system, are also best avoided.

Fresh paté

Paté comes with a (tiny) risk of listeria attached – official advice warns against meat, fish and even vegetable varieties, although you'll be fine with the potted or processed sort, such as those that come in a tin or are vacuum-packed.

Peanuts and peanut products

The FSA and the NHS want to wait for more evidence before issuing guidelines. At the time of writing, both bodies say that if you're pregnant and in a high-risk group (in other words, if you, or your baby's dad, have an allergy or an allergic condition such as eczema), you 'might want to' steer clear of peanuts and peanut products.

Pregnancy food myth busted

Eating peanuts won't give your baby a peanut allergy. Some doctors are beginning to suspect that, if anything, early exposure to allergens may be beneficial. You certainly don't need to avoid nuts if there is no history of allergy or allergic condition in your immediate family.

Barbecues and buffets

Bacteria breed quickly on food that's left uncovered in a warm place, so stick to food that's come fresh off the barbecue, and be selective when it comes to party spreads, steering clear of stuff such as prawns or cold meats, for example.

Chilled, unwrapped 'deli' foods such as cold meats, quiches, pies and salads; restaurant food; takeaways

The problem with these foods is that you can't be certain of their hygiene history. You *ought* to be fine with cold food from a reputable shop or establishment. Generally anything's okay if it's been (freshly) cooked or thoroughly heated through. So a slice of deli counter quiche is fine if you get it home and cook it in the oven for 15 minutes. Make sure takeaways are piping hot too.

Pocket tip 🍵

Whatever you do, try not to fret too much about food safety. Play it 100% safe if it feels the right thing to do, but don't let it become a source of high anxiety.

Tips for good food hygiene

- *Keep your kitchen clean.*
- *Wash your hands thoroughly before and after handling food.*
- *Thoroughly wash all fruit and vegetables.*
- *Defrost frozen meat and other foods thoroughly, preferably in the fridge.*
- *Cover food when in the fridge, and store raw and cooked products separately.*
- *Make sure all hot food is served piping.*
- *Make sure your fridge and freezer are at the correct temperatures (0–4°C for fridges, below −18°C for freezers).*
- *Chill or freeze food as soon as you get it home from the supermarket.*
- *Have separate chopping boards for raw foods and foods that are ready to eat.*
- *Eat food within the use-by dates.*
- *Keep pets out of the kitchen.*

FOOD CRAVINGS AND AVERSIONS

Pregnancy cravings – a yearning for a particular food, and more often than not a bizarre choice – are common. Some women also go off certain foods, most usually caffeine, alcohol and anything greasy or spicy. It's not clear why this happens, although there are theories – ranging from an evolutionary mechanism that ensures a pregnant woman gets what she needs (and avoids harmful food), to hormones or a psychological explanation.

What can I do about it?

They're generally harmless, although if your diet's very unhealthy as a result, you should curb them. The desire to eat a non-edible item could be more about texture than taste, so if you're affected, you may be able to get some relief from chewing on something crunchy but harmless, like ice.

Could it be serious?

Craving a non-food item is a psychological disorder known as **pica** and it could be serious if you eat too much of something that's inedible. Talk to your midwife or doctor about it if you're getting weird cravings and you're acting on them.

Pocket fact 🎲

Among the weird items pregnant women have been known to hanker for are sand, soil, soap, cigarette butts, matches, plaster, sandpaper and rubber.

Most common cravings

1. Chocolate
2. Ice cream
3. Sweets
4. Spicy food
5. Pickled onions
6. Tropical fruit
7. Curry
8. Doughnuts
9. Marmite

10. Peanut butter

11. Potatoes

12. Nuts

Weirdest cravings

1. Ice

2. Coal

3. Toothpaste

4. Sponges

5. Mud

6. Chalk

7. Laundry soap

8. Matches

9. Rubber

Strange craving combinations

- Pickles and peanut butter
- Marmite and ice cream
- Tuna and banana
- Fried eggs with mint sauce

Pocket fact 🎲

Pregnancy cravings affects 90% of women. This has risen dramatically, from 30% five decades ago.

Celebrity cravings

- Britney Spears: dirt
- Victoria Beckham: smoked salmon
- Minnie Driver: olives
- Jennifer Lopez: salsa, M&Ms and orange soda
- Gwen Stefani: tabasco
- Katie Holmes: cupcakes
- Davina McCall: Coca-Cola, sponges
- Myleen Klass: mangoes
- Amanda Holden: Guinness
- Catherine Zeta Jones: Branston pickle

Pocket tip ☕

Remember we're talking guidelines here, not laws; ultimately, the lifestyle you keep during pregnancy is down to you.

WATER

It's important to drink lots of water anyway, but when you're pregnant it's even more so. The World Health Organization advises that you should drink about 4.8 litres of water per day.

- It's easy to encourage yourself to meet this target by carrying around and drinking from a used water bottle (get the slightly bigger 750ml ones).
- Fill this up (and drink the contents) several times a day, and you're on your way.
- You can also get your daily fluid intakes from tea and coffee (remember your caffeine limits), fruit juices (dilute with water where possible) and milk (which will boost your calcium intake).

ALCOHOL

Pocket tip 🥤

If you know you've drunk alcohol before you found out you were pregnant, don't panic. Plenty of women have found themselves in this position. Chances are, you'll have caused no harm at all, although clearly it's a good idea to ease up on the drinking once you do know.

In 2007, the Government adopted the mantra that pregnant women, or women trying to conceive, should avoid alcohol altogether. However, there is no evidence that *light* drinking during pregnancy is harmful.

- If you want to stick to the recommended 'safe levels' of alcohol during pregnancy, aim for a maximum of 1–2 units a week, drunk just once or twice per week.

- When drinking, don't forget to count your units and the alcohol by volume (ABV) content of your glass (see the chart opposite).

- Don't binge drink – in other words, don't consume more than six units in one session. But don't worry if you were drunk on the odd occasion before you knew you were pregnant: you're unlikely to have caused any harm as it's *prolonged* heavy drinking that's most risky.

Pocket fact 🧱

It is recommended that drinking is to be particularly avoided during the first trimester, as that's when it may increase the risk of miscarriage.

What alcohol can do

Babies born to women who drink heavily during pregnancy – in other words, anyone drinking more than six units a day – are at significant risk of being born with a condition called Foetal Alcohol Syndrome (FAS), which can cause facial deformities, restricted growth and learning and behavioural difficulties. It will also increase your risk of:

- *Having a miscarriage (during the first trimester)*
- *Your baby's organs, nervous system and growth being affected*
- *Premature birth, or a low birth weight (which means your baby is more vulnerable to infections and other health problems)*
- *Your baby being more susceptible to illness later in life*
- *Suffering a stillbirth*

What's a unit?

Drink	ABV 12%	ABV 14%
Small (125ml) glass of wine	1.5 units	1.75
Standard (175ml) glass of wine	2.1	2.45
Large (250 ml) glass of wine	3	3.5

Drink	Unit
330ml bottle of 5% strength lager	1.7
Pint	2.8
25ml measure of spirit	1
35ml measure of spirit (usual amount served in pubs)	1.4
double (50ml) measure of spirit	2
275ml bottle of alcopop (ABV 5%)	1.4

Pocket tip 🍵

There's lots of information, plus a handy online units calculator, on the website of the Drinkaware Trust (www.drinkaware.co.uk).

CAFFEINE

It's thought that high levels of caffeine can increase the risk of low birth weight, making a baby more vulnerable to a range of health problems, and there's some evidence that links a very high consumption to miscarriage.

The Food Standards Agency (FSA), the Government's independent authority on food and nutrition, advises that 200mg of caffeine is a safe daily limit. This is around two mugs of instant coffee or one and a half of filter coffee. The FSA points out that if you occasionally have more than this you shouldn't worry, as 'the risks are likely to be very small'.

Caffeine is also found in tea, cola and other soft drinks, chocolate and certain medicines – see the list below.

How much caffeine does it contain?
- *Mug of instant coffee: 100mg*
- *Mug of fresh brewed or filter coffee: 140mg*
- *Mug of tea: 75mg*
- *Can of cola: 33mg*
- *Can of energy drink: 80mg*
- *50g bar of plain chocolate: 50mg*
- *50g bar of milk chocolate: 25mg*

Pocket tip 🖙

Many women are put off caffeine during morning sickness, which will help you avoid it no end.

HEALTHY EATING

It makes sense to eat as healthily as possible during pregnancy.

- You'll boost your immune system and have all the energy you need to meet the extra physical demands you're under.

- You'll also be less likely to pile on too many unwanted pounds.

- A good diet will help to boost the growth and development of your baby in a number of ways.

Pocket fact ▦

One recent study found that babies born to mums who ate lots of junk food are more likely to suffer health problems such as heart disease and diabetes later in their own lives.

Beware of 'eating for two'

The demands of pregnancy can be met with an average increase of no more than 200–300 calories a day, and that's only in the final trimester.

Putting on too much weight can put you at higher risk of developing conditions like pre-eclampsia (see p. 56) and gestational diabetes (see below), as well as putting extra strain on your body in general and raising the likelihood of difficulties during birth and labour more of a likelihood.

Pocket fact 🎲

*On average a woman will gain 22 pounds during pregnancy.
Within an hour of delivery she will lose 13.5 pounds and another
3.5 over the next 12 days. 6 weeks after giving birth she will
weigh about 18 pounds less than when she went into labour.*

Gestational diabetes

*Between 2% and 14% of women develop diabetes for the
first time in pregnancy, when it's known as gestational
diabetes. Being overweight, or putting on a lot of weight in
pregnancy, is a risk factor, as is a family history of diabetes,
and an ethnic background that's south Asian, black
Caribbean, or Middle Eastern. Your doctor will discuss this
and give you specific advice about how to look after yourself
and your baby.*

Tips for a healthy pregnancy diet

- **Fruit and veg:** Five portions a day is the minimum recommended. Remember that you can include lots of things that don't really feel like fruit and veg at all: fried mushrooms, baked beans, tomato-based pasta sauces, frozen sweetcorn, strawberries and cream, and fruit smoothies, for example.

- **Starchy foods (carbohydrates):** Aim for three or four servings of bread, rice, pasta or cereals a day, and plump for the healthier wholegrain or brown varieties whenever possible, which will help to ease constipation.

- **Protein:** Get at least two servings a day, in the form of meat, fish, eggs, beans or pulses.

Alternative sources of protein

Canned sardines (430mg per can)

Bread (83mg per two slices of white or wholemeal)

Baked beans (100mg per small can)

Nuts such as almonds (30mg per six nuts)

Green vegetables like broccoli (35mg per two florets)

Some products are fortified with extra calcium – certain cereals, orange juice, soya and tofu, for example – so it's always worth checking the labels.

- **Eat three meals a day:** As well as well-timed snacks to keep you going in between. Nutritious nibbles such as fresh and dried fruit, yoghurts and cheese, wholemeal bread or toast or a bowl of non-sugary cereal will be better for you than sweeties, cakes or crisps.

- **Calcium:** Really important for the growth and development of your baby's teeth and bones – get the recommended daily allowance (RDA) for an ordinary adult female, which is 700mg a day. That's a daily glass of milk (230mg), a pot of yoghurt (225mg) and a matchbox-sized piece of hard cheese (288mg).

- **Vitamin D:** This ensures your baby's bones develop well, and will also boost the content in your breast milk, which is already in production. Food sources include fortified margarines, eggs, meat and oily fish, but it's mostly provided by the sunlight we're exposed to (it's sometimes called 'the sunshine vitamin'). The Government recommends that *all* pregnant women take a 10 microgram (mcg) supplement of vitamin D daily.

- **Iron:** Requirements rise in pregnancy. Good sources of iron are red meat, leafy green vegetables such as spinach, watercress and broccoli, shellfish, eggs, dried fruits such as apricots or figs, nuts, pulses and beans, wholemeal bread, fortified breakfast cereals, and dark chocolate. Your doctor or midwife may suggest iron tablets if they're worried that you're seriously lacking it, but with some caution as they can cause constipation – already a prominent pregnancy side effect for many women.

- **Folic acid:** Taken prior to conception and during the first trimester, this can help to protect against neural tube defects such as spina bifida, a condition which can cause serious disabilities. You can get a certain amount from foods such as leafy green vegetables (spinach, sprouts or greens), citrus fruits and fortified breakfast cereals. However, official advice is to take a 400mcg supplement daily until your 12th week of pregnancy. Folic acid supplement tablets are readily available in chemists and supermarkets, and it's also included in most antenatal multivitamin supplements.

- **Omega 3 (or essential) fatty acids:** Reckoned to help boost your baby's brain and eyesight development. Oily fish is the best source – mackerel, sardines, kippers, salmon, fresh tuna. You can get a certain amount of omega 3 from nuts and seeds.

- **Drink lots:** Water's the healthiest drink around.

🛒 CIGARETTES 🛒

You know this one: if you smoke, give up now. If you smoke whilst pregnant, your risk of miscarriage and stillbirth increases by 26%, you're more likely to suffer some kind of complication, such as placental abruption (see p. 63), and there's more chance of your baby having a low birth weight or being born premature, and therefore more likely to suffer infections or other health problems. Once born, your baby will be more likely to have poor lung function, to suffer from difficulties in feeding, breathing problems like asthma, or chest and ear infections. Smoking is also one of the established risk factors for cot death – so stop now.

Pocket fact 🎓

According to NHS statistics, babies of mothers who smoke are, on average, about 7oz lighter at birth than others.

DOES IT MATTER THAT I SMOKED BEFORE I KNEW?

There's no need to worry if you smoked before you knew you were pregnant – the risks outlined above are linked to pregnancies where mums have smoked throughout. Stop in your first trimester and your baby will be okay.

🛒 MEDICINE 🛒

REGULAR MEDICATION

If you take regular medication for a chronic or long-term condition such as diabetes, asthma or epilepsy, make sure your doctor knows as soon as you know that you are pregnant. Don't stop taking your drugs without getting medical advice first, though.

OVER-THE-COUNTER MEDICATION

Pregnant women are generally advised to avoid over-the-counter medication unless it's really essential. However, you're fine to take the odd recommended dose of paracetamol and certain essential remedies such as Gaviscon, which tackles heartburn, are okay. If in doubt, ask your midwife, GP or the pharmacist before taking or applying anything, or give NHS Direct a call. Don't assume alternative or herbal remedies will be okay because they're 'natural' – some also have risks.

Pocket fact 🔢

The egg is the largest cell in the human body, while the sperm is the smallest. A single egg weighs the same as 175,000 sperm.

🍼 ACTIVITIES 🍼

What should be avoided in pregnancy? The bottom line is it's down to you. But here are some of the activities where a possible risk (in some cases, a *very* small one) has been identified:

IN THE HOME

- **Gardening:** There's a tiny risk of infection if you get soil with toxoplasmosis on your hands. Wear gardening gloves and wash your hands thoroughly when you're done.

- **Exposure to paints:** There's no firm evidence of danger either way. Modern, water-based household paints (like emulsions) are safe; however, the NHS advises that to be really safe, avoid painting in the first trimester. Don't use solvent-based paints, varnishes or brush cleaners at all. Avoid stripping any old paintwork too.

- **Household chemicals and cleaning products:** There's also no firm evidence. However, it makes sense to avoid powerful products such as pesticides and oven cleaners just to be on the safe side.

- **Contact with animals:** Cat poo has been found to harbour toxoplasmosis, so don't empty litter trays if you can help it, and use rubber gloves if you must. Bacteria is found in animal waste generally, so it's sensible to wash your hands after contact with pets.

Air travel

You can fly during an uncomplicated pregnancy, but it may make you feel more wretched during the first trimester, and there's a risk you'll go into labour near your due date. Some airlines don't allow pregnant travellers from 28 weeks. Policies vary, so always check before booking. The risk of DVT increases when you're pregnant, so move around lots during any flight and consider wearing support stockings.

EXERCISE

It's a good idea to keep up some kind of exercise throughout pregnancy if you can. It will:

- Boost your general fitness, flexibility and health
- Aid relaxation
- Reduce aches and pains
- Improve sleep
- Offset constipation
- Help prepare you for the physical demands of late pregnancy, labour and birth, and caring for a new baby

Pocket fact 🔡

Research suggests that if you keep fit during pregnancy, you're more likely to have a shorter labour time and fewer delivery complications.

If you're a fitness novice: Start something fairly gentle such as walking, swimming or organised sessions specifically designed for pregnancy, such as aqua-natal classes or antenatal yoga.

If you were already fit: Keep up the same level of activity as before for as long as you feel comfortable doing so.

Pocket tip 🖐

Do at least a little everyday activity where possible, and to keep up your 'pelvic floor'. See p. 45.

Tips for a healthy exercise regime

- Reconsider certain high-impact techniques that involve lots of fast twists and turns, such as step aerobics, as your body is more vulnerable to strain and injury.

- Reduce the risk of injury by making sure you do warm-up and cool-down exercises either side of a workout.

- A decent pair of trainers, where trainers are required, is also important.

- Drink plenty of water before, during and after exercise.

- Wear appropriate clothing.

- Don't work out in very hot and humid weather.

- Avoid overexerting yourself.

Pocket tip 👌

How much is overexertion? Use the 'talk test' to give a good indi-cation of how your body's coping: you should be able to continue a conversation whilst exercising without catching your breath.

What sort of exercise is suitable?

- **Aerobic (cardiovascular) exercise, such as power-walking, running, dancing and low-impact aerobic classes** is fine during pregnancy – if that's what your body is used to.

- **Walking** – a great pregnancy exercise, do this if you've never done aerobic exercise before. Try an ordinary (but brisk) pace.

- **Swimming** – gives your heart and muscles a gentle workout. It's highly recommended in pregnancy as the buoyancy of the water will support you and your bump and it's low impact, and therefore unlikely to leave you injured. However, the leg action of a breast stroke can put pressure on the lower back and pelvis, particularly if you tend to swim with your head out of the water, so if you're suffering from pain in those areas you may be better off sticking to front or back crawl.

- **Yoga** or **pilates** – strength conditioning exercises like these can improve your muscle tone and flexibility, but won't improve your cardiovascular fitness (ideally, you'd do a bit of both sorts of exercise). They're great in pregnancy, as they can help to strengthen the 'core' muscles of your pelvic floor and lower abdomen, and they're particularly relaxing ways of exercising. Look for one designed for antenatal requirements.

Pocket tip 🗇

Take the stairs: *If you lack the energy and motivation to exercise, aim to at least fit some sort of activity into your life so you don't really notice it. The best way to do this is by taking the stairs instead of the lift whenever you're presented with the choice, and by walking everywhere you possibly can.*

Gentle strength conditioning exercises you can do at home

Pelvic tilts

- Stand with your shoulders and bottom against a wall, keeping your knees soft.

- Tilt your pelvis, so that your back flattens against the wall, and hold for about four seconds, continuing to breathe.

- Repeat up to 10 times.

'The cat'

- Get down on all fours with your hands under your shoulders and gently hold in your tummy, so that your back is flat.

- Now draw in your tummy and tilt the pelvis so that your bottom tucks under, your back rounds upwards and your head curls underneath.

- Hold for a few seconds before returning to the neutral position, then repeat.

Pelvic floor exercises

Pelvic floor exercises done regularly throughout pregnancy and after birth can make a real difference in preventing leaking urine when coughing, sneezing, exercising or laughing – caused by your pelvic floor muscles supporting a giant uterus for nine months and neglecting their other duties. They're not difficult and you can do them any time and any place – at your desk, watching telly, whilst washing up, etc.

- First, identify where your pelvic floor muscles are. The best way to do this is to imagine you're trying to stop weeing mid-flow (don't try this when you are actually weeing, as it can cause urinary tract infections to do so), or gripping a tampon with your vagina. Don't be tempted to tighten your tummy, buttocks or thighs, as these aren't the muscles you're looking for.

- Try squeezing and releasing the muscles quickly, repeating up to 10 times.

- Then squeeze slowly, trying to hold the muscles tight for up to 10 seconds before relaxing.

- Repeat this 10 times, too.

- Ideally, you should do both sets of squeezes four to six times a day.

Pocket tip ☞

Put little coloured stickers in various places throughout your home and in the car, as reminders to do a few squeezes when you see them. Nobody else needs to know what they're for.

When you shouldn't exercise

Generally speaking, you should stop exercising and seek prompt advice if you experience one or more of the following symptoms.

- Dizziness or feeling faint

- Headache

- Shortness of breath on exertion

- Difficulty in getting your breath whilst exercising

- Pain or palpitations in your chest

- Pain in your abdomen, back or pubic area, or in your pelvic girdle

- Weakness in your muscles

- Pain or swelling in one or both legs

- Painful uterine contractions

- Fewer movements from your baby

- Leakage of your amniotic fluids

- Bleeding

OTHER ACTIVITIES

- **Mountaineering and hot air ballooning:** The high altitudes involved mean a change in oxygen levels that could potentially trigger a miscarriage. Scuba diving is also not a good idea because of potential decompression sickness and an increased risk of miscarriage.

- **Extreme sports such as hang-gliding, rock-climbing, skydiving and bungee jumping:** Don't do this – for fairly obvious safety reasons!

- **Theme parks:** Rapid stops and starts can damage the womb, and are best avoided. Water slides should be enjoyed with caution – most display a warning notice to steer clear if you're expecting.

🛒 OUT AND ABOUT 🛒

STOP TOUCHING MY BELLY!

One thing's going to happen to your body for sure: before too long, you'll be the proud owner of a lovely big, firm bump. Most women find that their big bellies prove a draw to all sorts of people (random strangers included), keen to stroke, poke and generally comment on it. Depending on the mood you're in, this can be one of the more irritating factors about pregnancy.

- Try to breathe deeply and keep smiling when you come into contact with a 'prodder'.
- If you can't handle it, smile politely, take a step back and walk away.
- Make sure you set boundaries you're happy with amongst your family and friends. The likelihood is you won't mind them touching it, as much as complete strangers, but at least you can be honest with them.

Pocket fact 🎲

Babies recognise their mother's voice at birth but it takes 14 days for them to recognise their father's.

TRAVELLING WITH BABY

Getting a seat on public transport is one of the great trials of pregnancy. Ironically, you won't get offered one when you might feel you need it most, in the first trimester, and for most of the second your fellow travellers will probably be so worried that you're simply fat, rather than pregnant, they won't want to ask. Sadly, even being very obviously pregnant is no guarantee that someone will do the decent thing.

Tips for pregnant travel

- Try to avoid the worst of the rush hour. Even 15–30 minutes could make all the difference.

- Once you're showing, unbutton your coat and stick your belly out, so there's no doubt that you're in the family way.

- Be bold. Ask outright for a seat if you feel you need one.

- Get a big, bold *Baby on Board* badge. You can get these from most London Underground stations, or online from pregnancy websites.

- Don't leave home without a snack and a bottle of water in your bag. You may need sustenance if you feel faint or poorly.

DRIVING WHILE PREGNANT

If you drive a lot, make sure you're as comfortable as you can be in the driving seat.

- If your back hurts, you might get a bit of relief from a small cushion supporting your lower back.

- Break the journey up to stretch your legs if it's a long one.

Once you've got a reasonable-sized bump, consider investing in a 'bump belt', a cushioned strap that can be easily attached to, and detached from, your seat belt, keeping it in a position underneath your bump and allowing a safer and more comfortable ride for you and your baby.

🍼 INTIMACY AND SEX 🍼
DURING PREGNANCY

Sex can become a little scarce in the nine months that follow conception.

- It's very normal for women to have little sex drive in the first trimester, as sickness and exhaustion take their toll; a more active second trimester, as you begin to feel human again; and a return to the drought during the third. It doesn't always work that way, of course.

- Some women find their sex drive remains unchanged through pregnancy. Others are virtually celibate for the duration.

- It's totally normal for one or both halves of a couple to go off sex for some reason during pregnancy, and that's fine. Sex lives *do* tend to get put on hold when you become parents and, fortunately, they almost always come back again.

- If things are lacking in the bedroom department, it's a really good idea to talk about why, if you can, and to make sure that there are plenty of kisses, cuddles and touching to make up for it. It's very easy to feel rejected when your partner doesn't want to have sex with you, even if they do have a damn good excuse, so it's important to make sure the 'unwilling' party lets the other one know they still care.

- Sex can be used to bring on labour — see p. 143 for more on this.

Pregnancy sex worries busted
A handful of myths about sex in pregnancy tend to persist. But you can rest assured:

- ***The baby won't get squashed.*** *He's very well cushioned in his amniotic sac and will be completely untroubled.*
- ***The baby has no idea you are having sex.*** *He might hear you, and he might kick and move around a bit, but it won't scar him for life.*
- ***Your partner's penis – however big it may be – will never ever make contact with your baby.*** *The angle of the vagina means that there's no way his penis will bump the baby. It's anatomically impossible.*

LOOKING AFTER YOUR RELATIONSHIP

It's not just the physical side of your love life that's affected by pregnancy. It can be a challenging time emotionally, too.

- The best thing you can do to keep your love for each other ticking over healthily during pregnancy is to talk to each other. Let your partner know what's going on with you and your body – he won't understand completely but you can give him an idea.

- Talking's a two-way street of course: so make sure you extend an ear to him, too.

- If you're arguing more than usual, be sure to kiss and make up before things get out of hand.

- Pencil in as many slots as possible to spend with each other: make a date with each other one of your main priorities.

- Discuss your plans for the birth, and for parenthood, and talk about the changing phases of your pregnancy by all means.

- Sometimes it's a good idea to put the whole pregnancy/baby thing out of the equation for a while, and talk about something completely different.

- Try to give each other a bit of space where necessary. Encourage him to see his friends, and meet up with yours too, even if you don't feel like it sometimes.

Above all, try to keep in mind that pregnancy is a temporary phase in any couple's shared lifetime. Most people find that – ultimately – pregnancy and parenthood bring them closer, not further apart.

Pocket tip ☕

If your relationship really seems in trouble, it would be a good idea to thrash things out before the baby's arrival. You might want to consider some couples counselling through an organisation such as Relate.

'Pregnancy makes you feel more like a woman than you've ever felt.'

Angelina Jolie

🍼 PREGNANCY AND WORK 🍼

The subject of when to leave work confuses many women, who don't know their rights or their options. Here, we give you the simple facts, so that you can make an informed decision.

> *Pocket fact* 🔡
>
> *In most cases maternity leave won't begin until a month or so before your due date, if not later.*

TELLING YOUR BOSS

- You must tell your boss before you're 25 weeks' pregnant. In fact, it's sensible to let them know as early as you can, so that any necessary plans can be put into place and your risk assessment (see below) can be carried out.

- You need to let your boss know when your baby is due and when you want your maternity leave and pay to start (see below). You might be required to do this in writing.

- You'll also need to present them with your maternity certificate (form MATB1), which your midwife will give to you after you're 21 weeks' pregnant and which confirms your due date.

- Your employer must then give you written confirmation of your return date within 28 days (and unless you tell them otherwise, they must assume you're going to take your full maternity leave entitlement of 12 months).

- You *can* tell your boss if you know for sure you want to come back before the full entitlement period is up (and you can change your mind, as long as you give eight weeks' notice of your revised return date). Many women choose to wait and see how they feel.

The attitude of your boss and your colleagues can really affect how you cope with your career during pregnancy. Having a supportive boss can make the world of difference.

KNOW YOUR RIGHTS

What follows is only a basic guide to your legal rights as a pregnant employee. It's a complex subject and one woman's entitlements can vary from another's. The best source of basic information is the Directgov website (www.direct.gov.uk).

Maternity leave

- All pregnant employees have the right to take up to 12 months off work – it doesn't matter how long you've worked for a company or what your hours are.

- The first 26 weeks of maternity leave is called ordinary maternity leave (OML). You can begin OML up to 11 weeks before your baby is due – the medical view is that eight weeks is a sensible time to take off before your due date; however, most women prefer to waddle in to work for as long as humanly possible, giving them more time off with their baby once he's born.

- If you have to take time off work because of medical issues related to your pregnancy in the four weeks before your due date, you're automatically considered to have begun your OML.

- If you give birth before your planned leave kicks off, your maternity leave will be considered to have started from then on.

Pocket fact ▦

You should still be entitled to any contractual benefits you might get (gym membership, for example) during your leave and your company must continue to make contributions to your pension if they do that already.

You're also entitled to take any holiday that builds up in your maternity period — lots of women choose to use this to boost their total amount of maternity leave.

Maternity pay

If you were working for your employer when you became pregnant, and you're earning more than £90 a week, you qualify for Statutory Maternity Pay (SMP). Paid through your employer, you get (at the time of writing):

- 90% of your average pay for the first six weeks
- £117.18 per week (or 90% of your average earnings if it's less than this) for a further 33 weeks.

So if you *do* decide to take the full year's maternity leave you're entitled to, the last three months of your maternity leave will be unpaid.

Some companies have their own maternity pay schemes in place, and you may find that your employer has a more generous rate of maternity pay than the statutory rate (usually on the basis that you'll return to work for a certain period when your maternity leave is over — and if you decide not to go back to work you may have to pay some of it back).

You may not be entitled to get SMP if you weren't employed for the qualifying period or earning the qualifying amount, if you're a casual worker, or if you're self-employed or unemployed.

In these cases, you can usually claim Maternity Allowance instead, which is £117.18 per week for 39 weeks, or 90% of your average pay if it's less than this. You'll need a claim form for this (MA1), which you can download from the Department for Work and Pensions website (www.dwp.gov.uk).

Your partner's paternity rights

Your partner may qualify for up to two weeks' paternity leave with statutory paternity pay – he may even work for a company that offers an enhanced scheme with a better deal. He'll need to give notice of his intentions at least 15 weeks before your due date.

Time off for antenatal care

Your employer must let you have time off for anything that counts as an antenatal care appointment – and this could even include something like a relaxation or parentcraft class if your midwife or GP has advised you to attend.

Keeping in touch

You can spend up to 10 days in your workplace, for which you can be paid, during maternity leave if you want to. Known as 'Keeping in Touch' days, you can keep up with what's going on at work and maintain links with your colleagues. These are by no means compulsory, though, from either your point of view or your boss's.

Equally, your employer is entitled to make 'reasonable contact' with you while you're away, if they need to refer to you about a work matter that just can't wait. But he or she cannot demand you go in to work for any reason – that's down to you.

Returning to work after your maternity leave

- You must give your employer 28 days' notice if you plan to return to work before the end of ordinary maternity leave (in other words, during the first 26 weeks of your year's entitlement), or eight weeks' notice if you plan to go back during additional maternity leave (ie during the second 26 weeks).

- If you go back before the ordinary maternity leave period is up, you're entitled to go back to the same job you had before leaving to have your baby.

- If you go back during your additional maternity leave, you should either get your old job back or be offered something else where the terms and conditions are just as good.

- If you decide not to go back to work at all, you have to give your employer whatever notice period your contract demands. You won't have to pay back any SMP – but if your company has paid you more than the statutory level under enhanced maternity benefits, they could ask you to pay all, or some, of it back.

- You may also decide you want to request a return to work with shorter hours or a more flexible set-up. There's a bit more about this below.

Your health and safety

By law, your employer must do whatever it takes to protect your health and safety during pregnancy. They must carry out a specific risk assessment based on your individual needs. Obviously it depends on what your job is, but some potential workplace risks are:

- Lifting or carrying heavy loads
- Standing or sitting for long lengths of time
- Exposure to infectious diseases, lead, hazardous chemicals, radioactive material, excessive noise, extremes of temperature, or to shock and vibration

- Work-related stress
- Workstations and posture
- Long working hours
- Mental and physical fatigue
- Threat of violence

If there *is* a risk and your working conditions or hours can't be adjusted to protect you from it, your employer must find you suitable alternative work on the same terms and conditions, and if that can't be done, you should be suspended from work on paid leave for as long as is necessary.

Pocket tip ☞

If you're concerned that your needs aren't being met, and you've talked to your company to no avail, contact an organisation such as Citizens Advice, ACAS, or the Health and Safety Executive (HSE) for advice.

WHEN YOU'RE THE BOSS

If you run your own company or work for yourself, it will be down to you to decide how long you go on working and how much time you take off with your baby. Ask yourself some questions: can you survive on maternity allowance and, if so, for how long? You'll also be responsible for taking care of yourself and ensuring your own health and safety.

Coping with stress

If you do a job where anxiety levels are high, you may quite reasonably worry about the effect it could have on your baby. Fortunately, unborn babies will generally be unaffected by their mother's stress.

TIRED ALL THE TIME?

Plain old exhaustion is one of the hardest things to deal with while working throughout pregnancy.

- During the first trimester surging hormones can cause an overpowering urge to sleep – and during the third, you might just lose the will to move altogether.

- If you're struggling to get through the day, take a short lunch-time 'power' nap if need be (a snooze of about 15–20 minutes is ideal – any more than that and you may feel worse than when you started).

- In theory employers have a duty to provide a place for you to rest, if possible, although in reality it may not be practical. At the very least, a chair and a desk or other surface for you to lay your head down may be better than nothing.

BEING COMFORTABLE AT WORK

- If you're on your feet, wear the most comfortable shoes you can bear.

- If you're sitting down all day, be sure to take a short break from your workstation for a few moments, preferably at least once or twice an hour.

- Make certain your desk and chair are positioned to give you maximum comfort, too – you should ask for a new set-up if your existing one doesn't give you enough space or is causing you discomfort that could otherwise be avoided.

- Make sure your chair is high enough. Your feet should be flat on the floor with your hips slightly higher than your knees. Raise your feet if necessary with help from a box or stool.

- Your computer screen should be positioned directly in front of you.

- Give your spine support with a small cushion or rolled up towel placed between the chair and the small of your back.

- Armrests can help you get out of your chair.

- Take regular breaks. Get up and move around for a couple of minutes, at least a couple of times an hour.

- Don't cross your legs – it will twist your spine and can affect the circulation.

- Sit up straight, but with relaxed shoulders.

- Try to keep your pelvis tilted slightly upwards while you sit.

- Don't forget that your needs may change as your bump gets bigger and sitting becomes increasingly uncomfortable.

When morning sickness takes over

Some managers may be reluctant to make allowances for severe morning sickness. But the law says they cannot discriminate against you in these circumstances – time off for pregnancy-related problems should be considered no different from any general sick leave (except if it happens in the last four weeks before you're due to start your leave, in which case your employer is entitled to clock you off for maternity leave as of then).

If you do need to take time off sick because you're ill in pregnancy and you get any grief about it, get a note from your midwife and GP, and stand firm. Remember, you cannot be threatened with discipline or sacking just for taking time off if you're ill during pregnancy.

IF YOUR BOSS IS HORRIBLE

Even if your manager is technically playing the game, you may still be suffering from more resentful attitudes or a lack of support.

- Try to rise above any less-than-helpful mindsets by focusing on doing your job as best you can, thinking about your baby and reminding yourself that it's a short-term period in your life with an end goal that overrides everything else.

- Remind yourself that the law is on your side: if you're not happy with the way you're being treated, swot up on your rights and don't be afraid to share that information with your boss if you need to.

THINKING ABOUT THE FUTURE

Although you may not be ready yet to make a decision about what the future holds for you, work-wise, it's something to think about. Many women change their minds once they've had their baby. Have a general game plan in mind – but remain open-minded, too.

If you know or think that you're going back to work at some point, you will need to sort out some reliable childcare. It's never too early to be looking into this, so start looking around your area for what is convenient to you and what you can afford.

REQUESTING FLEXIBLE WORKING

Lots of women find that returning to work, but on a more flexible or part-time basis than before, gives them the work–life balance they're looking for. There's no law that says you *must* be given flexible work if you want it; however, anyone who's been with an employer for 26 weeks who has a child aged under six (dads, too) is entitled to *request* it – and their manager *must* give it 'serious consideration'. You've nothing to lose by asking.

7

PREPARING FOR THE BIRTH

Whilst you can never really know what birth's like until you've actually been through it, you *can* help yourself be ready for it by doing your homework. The important thing is to bear in mind is that where birth's concerned – particularly your first – nothing's guaranteed. So when it comes to planning yours, keep an open mind.

Raspberry leaf

Taking a regular dose of this herbal remedy in the last six to eight weeks before your baby's birth is reckoned to help stimulate the uterus and encourage a shorter labour. There's no scientific evidence to back this view, but some women swear by it. You can take it in one of two forms: either in a tablet, or by infusing the dried leaves in hot water to make a tea – both are available from health food shops. Don't take raspberry leaf tea any earlier in pregnancy, though.

🛒 WHERE YOU'RE GOING 🛒
TO GIVE BIRTH

There are three basic options when it comes to where you're going to give birth:

- Consultant-led hospital unit
- Midwife-led (or GP-led) unit
- Home birth

Once you've made the decision about where to give birth, you don't have to stick to it. You're entitled to change your mind at any point.

CONSULTANT-LED HOSPITAL UNIT

The majority of women have their babies in a consultant-led hospital maternity unit.

- Here you can access all pain relief drugs and any special equipment that's required, there'll always be an obstetrician on call if needed during the pregnancy or birth, and you'll be in the best place should an emergency arise.

- You'll generally be offered a chance to take a look around the maternity unit once you're booked in. Use it as a chance to ask questions and familiarise yourself with the layout.

- You can also find out what potentially useful equipment there is available: for instance, a birthing pool, aids such as birthing balls, comfy cushions, or bean bags, and a CD or cassette player.

- Delivery rooms these days tend to be more comfortable and better equipped for birth than they used to be. But if not, you might be able to bring what you need from home.

Pocket tip 🗇

A 7 week old embryo has the same features and internal organs as an adult but is only an inch long.

MIDWIFE-LED UNIT

In some areas, and providing you're not at high risk of some complication arising during birth, you may also be offered the option of having your baby in the more 'homely' setting of a midwife-led maternity unit, sometimes called a GP-led unit, or a birthing or birth centre.

- These usually operate independently, but some are attached to hospitals and may even work alongside consultant-led units.

- Here the focus is more likely to be on a relaxed and natural birthing experience.

- Birthing centres are well equipped with the things that make natural birth more of a possibility: water pools, for example, and staffed by midwives who'll usually be passionately in favour of natural birth.

- But there won't be an obstetrician or anaesthetist immediately to hand (so, no epidurals available – see p. 116), and there are no facilities for surgery, or for special baby care, which is why you'll be discouraged from booking in at this kind of centre if you're considered high risk.

GIVING BIRTH AT HOME

This is still fairly unusual (about one in 50 babies in the UK are born at home) but is becoming less so. In theory, this option is open to all women, although in reality there are still some areas where you might be discouraged, or even told outright it won't be possible, with staff shortages or cutbacks usually given the blame.

- You're likely to be discouraged from having a home birth if there's any complicating factor that means you'd be safer giving birth in a hospital. However, what constitutes a risk could vary according to the opinion of who you're talking to.

- The advantages to home birth are that there's less likelihood of needing intervention, a more comfortable, private and peaceful environment, and the possibility of a much calmer, more relaxing experience than a hospital birth.

- You will also be under the care of just one or two community midwives who'll stick with you throughout the whole experience, rather than subject to the changing shift patterns of the average maternity unit.

- Bear in mind that your pain relief options will be limited.

- You also have to accept that, in certain situations – if there are complications – you will have to go into hospital anyway.

- You can hire an independent midwife, which is a pretty expensive option (fees range from £1,500 to £4,000) but does ensure you do get one-to-one care.

Pocket fact 🔡
Cindy Crawford had a home birth after a 17-hour labour.

🍼 BIRTH PLANS 🍼

Some people are sceptical about birth plans because they're very often scrapped once the realities of birth happen. They are useful, though, but not compulsory. Look at your birth plan as a tool to make you think through the options, not as a rigid plan.

Pocket tip ☞

Make sure it's typed or written neatly so that the midwife can actually make sense of it. And let your antenatal care team know your thoughts – they'll be able to let you know if there's anything about your personal circumstances that might be relevant.

What to include

- Pain relief you might want – and any that you'd quite like to avoid.

- Who your birth partner's going to be.

- What sort of positions you're keen to try out and whether you'd like to remain active if possible.

- Whether you'd like to give the birthing pool a go, if one is available.

- Any desire you may have to avoid certain procedures – induction, or an episiotomy – if at all possible.

- If one method of intervention is preferable to you over another, for instance if you think a vacuum extraction delivery would be less of a concern than one involving forceps.

- Whether or not you're happy to have an injection to speed up the delivery of the placenta.

- If your partner is keen to cut the umbilical cord.

- How you plan to feed your baby. If you want to breastfeed, the midwife will probably help you to try straight away.

Pocket tip 🛒

For some women, a birth plan may amount to nothing more than the following phrase: 'I am happy for you to do whatever it takes to help me give birth to my baby safely.' And that's absolutely fine.

🛒 PAIN RELIEF 🛒

In the vast majority of births, pain relief of some kind is used. And there are a few options to consider. A minority of women make it through birth without, either through choice or because circumstances dictate.

ENTONOX (GAS AND AIR)

What is it? Gas and air (50% oxygen and 50% nitrous oxide) that you breathe in through a mask.

When can I have some? Any time during labour and birth, and whenever you feel the need. Since it also comes in portable canisters, it's the one form of pain relief you can rely on if you're giving birth at home. You'll also be able to use it if you're giving birth in water, unlike most other forms of pain relief.

Is it any good? It's one of the least powerful forms of pain relief for birth, but it can certainly take the edge off. It can take up to a minute for the effects to kick in, so it's best to take it when you feel a contraction coming.

Are there any drawbacks? Gas and air creates a sort of 'high' that can render you a bit woozy (a bit like being drunk). Otherwise it has no adverse effects and is safe for you and your baby.

TENS MACHINE

What is it? A TENS (transcutaneous electrical nerve stimulation) machine is a little box that emits electrical pulses through four wires and four sticky pads, which you fix to your back. It works by intercepting pain signals to your brain and by stimulating the release of endorphins, the body's natural pain-busting hormones.

When can I have some? You can wire yourself up to your TENS machine as early as you like, and as it takes up to an hour for your body to respond you should make sure you get it on in good time. You'll probably want to take it off towards the later stages of labour, as it's unlikely to help with very strong contractions.

Is it any good? Opinions vary – some women find them helpful, others say they're not particularly effective.

What are the drawbacks? If you turn the voltage up too high by mistake, the pulse can be uncomfortably strong. You won't be able to get a back massage, either, as the pads will get in the way. TENS machines aren't routinely available in maternity units – although some NHS trusts lend them out – so if you want one you'll probably need to buy or hire it. They're available from a whole range of places, including specialist companies (just Google 'TENS') and from big shops such as Boots or Mothercare. Expect to pay between £20 and £30 to hire, and around £50–£60 to buy.

PAINKILLING DRUGS SUCH AS PETHIDINE, MEPTID AND DIAMORPHINE

What is it? These painkilling drugs are usually given via an injection in the thigh or bum, or occasionally directly into the bloodstream. Midwives are able to administer them, so there'll be no need to call in a doctor if you want some. Pethidine is the most widely used, while Meptid and Diamorphine are available only in some units.

When can I have it? At any point, except when you're coming close to the pushing stage. You may be able to arrange to have Pethidine at a home birth, but many midwives would be reluctant to administer it in these circumstances because of the risks to the baby.

Is it any good? Reports from women vary – some say they were effective, others that they were little or no help in relieving the pain, although they usually make it easier to rest and relax between contractions.

What are the drawbacks? They can make you feel very drowsy, dizzy or sick.

Pocket fact 🔡

Around a quarter of women have an epidural during their first birth.

EPIDURAL

What is it? An anaesthetic injection into the spine, which numbs the nerve supply that serves the uterus and cervix, giving complete, and fast, relief from pain.

When can I have some? As soon as the pains start to become intolerable. The effects last for several hours, but you may need 'top-up' doses. However, it's best if it's worn off when the time comes to start pushing, as you'll be able to do so much more effectively if you've got sensation down there. Epidurals have to be administered by an anaesthetist, so you may have to wait if he or she is busy elsewhere in the hospital – women have been known to wait so long for one that it's too late. In some hospitals, you might not get one at all if it's the middle of the night. You won't be able to have one at home, or in a birthing centre, which are staffed solely by midwives.

Is it any good? Very effective indeed, usually.

What are the drawbacks? You can end up numb to your toes, and that means you can't get up and walk around. An epidural can weaken contractions and the lack of sensation can make it harder to push. You'll need a drip in your arm, as a precaution in case your blood pressure drops and you need to be given fluid urgently, and your baby will also need to be continuously monitored. You're likely to have a catheter, too (a tube going into your bladder, to remove wee), as you can't feel whether your bladder is full or not, all of which means your mobility will be restricted. Sometimes there can be side effects, such as a fever, shaking, headache or backache.

ALTERNATIVE METHODS

The jury's out on just how much these treatments can help and, if they do at all, how they work. However, the fact remains that lots of women find one – or several, used in conjunction – helpful in the early stages of labour.

Water

Sinking into a birthing pool full of warm water is widely reported to be very effective method of natural pain relief. Women who've used it with success say that water can aid comfort and relaxation, and often claim it helped them towards a 'calm' and 'peaceful' experience. Once in the water, you won't be able to have any other pain relief apart from gas and air.

Acupuncture

This ancient Chinese therapy involves the insertion of fine needles into various points of the body, which, it's said, stimulate the energy channels and release endorphins, the body's natural painkilling hormones. If you decide it could be for you, you'll need to find a qualified private practitioner.

Aromatherapy

Oils can be administered in a variety of ways, for example with massage, or through inhalation from a burner or vaporiser, or drops of oil infused on a hankie. Some oils are more suitable than others for labour. Do consult a trained aromatherapist for advice. It's unlikely that aromatherapy in itself will do very much to boost your pain threshold. But it may well aid relaxation and therefore help you cope better in the early part of labour.

Reflexology

This involves massaging particular points of the feet and is said to work in a similar way to acupuncture, by tapping into the body's energy channels and helping to release naturally occurring painkillers and reducing anxiety. Again, you will need to find a qualified practitioner to help you.

Hypnosis

Hypnobirthing is based on the theory that fear causes tension and tension makes pain worse, and involves putting the mind into a deep state of relaxation. To learn the techniques, you'll need to find a registered therapist – and you'll have to practise before the birth. There are also CDs available that claim to teach self-hypnosis.

Massage

Get your partner to gently rub your shoulders to help reduce tension, or focus on the lower back, where the pain of contractions is often most intense. Ask him to use long, slow, rhythmic and fairly firm strokes or circles with his fingers or the palm of his hands.

Breathing techniques

Slow, rhythmic, deep breathing can help you relax during labour and you're more likely to cope with pain if you relax into it, rather than tense up.

- *Focus on a two-syllable word, for instance 'relax', and repeat it in your mind in time to your breathing – 'reeeeee', as you breathe in, and 'laaax', as you breathe out. (You can use any word, but relax seems a good option.)*
- *Also try counting whilst you breathe or, more simply, breathing in through your nose and out through your mouth.*
- *Trying to keep your shoulders loose and relaxed can help reduce tension, too.*

Your birth partner can get involved and help out by breathing along with you. As with other natural ways of coping with pain, you might find that deep breathing only takes you a certain distance.

🍼 YOUR BIRTH PARTNER 🍼

Most women want to bring someone along to hold their hand when they have a baby. Usually this will be your other half, if you have one. But not everyone wants to take their man into the labour room with them and not every man is keen to go. You could also have:

- A close female friend or relative with you
- Hired professional help in the form of a 'doula' – these are trained birth assistants who offer practical and emotional support

What your birth partner can do in advance of the birth

- Be sure he knows where the maternity unit phone number is.
- Take responsibility for the journey to hospital by making sure the car's shipshape and full of petrol, and that he knows the route. Check out the geography and cost of parking at the hospital.
- Make sure your bag is put in the car.
- Have a clear idea of what your hopes for labour and birth are. Get him to read the birth plan – but consult you during labour to make sure you still want to go with it.

🛒 PLANNED CAESAREAN SECTION 🛒

Pocket fact 🎲

Whether planned or not, Caesareans are relatively common: they account for around 20% of births in this country.

You may find out in advance of your due date that you're going to have a Caesarean section (sometimes shortened to c-section). It'll be known as a 'planned' or 'elective' Caesarean (rather than an emergency one). There are a number of reasons why an obstetrician may want to pencil in a c-section for a first-time birth. For instance:

- If you're suffering from pre-eclampsia (see p. 56).

- If it's been found or is suspected that your baby's head is too big to pass through your pelvis (known as cephalopelvic disproportion).

- If your baby is in a breech (bottom first) or transverse (sideways) position and attempts to turn him around have failed (see p. xx). (Although, it is possible to have a breech baby vaginally – see p. xx.)

- If you're expecting twins or more, since there are more likely to be complications (although in some cases it is quite possible to give birth to twins in the normal way. Any more than two babies, though, and you'll be very strongly advised to go with the c-section). For more, see the box on twin deliveries, below.

- If you have placenta praevia (see p. 62) – in other words, the placenta is partially or completely blocking the exit to the womb.

- If you have an infection, for instance genital herpes, that could be passed to the baby during a vaginal birth.

- If you have a chronic medical condition such as heart disease or diabetes that would make the strain of a normal labour potentially dangerous for you.

Doctors won't automatically carry out a Caesarean section without a good reason. The doctor *must* consult you and explain his reasoning, though, outline any risks and benefits, and will need your consent. There's more on Caesareans on p. xx.

Pocket fact 🔡

Tokophobia is a genuine fear of childbirth.

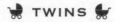 TWINS

Some doctors will routinely recommend a planned Caesarean section if you're having twins because there's more risk of complications arising – but policies and attitudes vary, depending on who's looking after you. However, it's quite possible for twins to be born in the normal way – and around half are.

Twins are usually born slightly earlier than most babies, at around 37 weeks, because there's less room in the womb for them to move around, which means they're smaller on average than singleton babies and so a bit more vulnerable.

Pocket fact

The Khamsa identical quadruplets born in 2002 are the most babies to be born from a single egg fertilised by a single sperm. The girls are genetically identical and research suggests identical quadruplets only occur once in 11 million births.

PREMATURE BABIES

If your baby is born before 37 weeks, his birth is considered premature – about one baby in every 10 makes their appearance before this point.

There are many reasons why your baby might be born early:

- You've gone into labour spontaneously.

- Your doctor has induced you or carried out a c-section because he feels it would be risky not to.

- Twins or more are likely to make an earlier than normal exit, since it becomes rather a squeeze when you're sharing a womb in the late stages.

- Women older than 35 are slightly more at risk of premature birth.

- Premature rupture of the membranes (in other words, your waters breaking early) is a common cause and this can be triggered by a number of things, including infection or excess amniotic fluid.

Often there'll be warning signs that premature birth is a likelihood, which a midwife or doctor will pick up during your routine antenatal checks.

Pocket fact 🎲

One in three premature babies are delivered by c-section because of an increased risk of complications.

Special care babies, even those born quite some weeks before they're due, have a good chance of survival these days because the care and equipment available in special care baby units is so advanced.

Recent figures show that babies born as early as 23 weeks have a 20% chance of survival, whilst at 25 weeks they have a 67% chance of survival. By 32 weeks, almost all babies will survive without any major health problems.

Parents are well served by Bliss, the charity for babies born too soon, too small or too sick.

🍼 ANTENATAL CLASSES 🍼

Your antenatal classes will usually begin somewhere between 6 and 12 weeks before your due date. They're a good opportunity to pick up some tips about stuff like pain relief and can be a useful way to force your other half to take an interest.

SIGNING UP

Antenatal classes tend to get booked up very quickly, so sign up now – especially for those run by the National Childbirth Trust (NCT).

- Fees for NCT courses range from £90 to £240 depending on where you live, although there are opportunities for subsidies

- If you can't get into an NCT class, or can't afford to pay, your midwife or doctor will tell you about the NHS classes available in your area.

THE CLASSES

As well as being a useful way to get the information you need about pregnancy and to help you prepare emotionally and practically for the birth, antenatal classes can be a good place to meet other prospective parents – you may even forge some long-term friendships.

- NHS antenatal classes (often called parentcraft classes) will be run by a midwife and are usually pretty basic. Their availability and scheduling can also be a bit hit and miss, as they tend to be subject to funding and staff cuts.

- NCT classes are run by specially trained teachers and take place in small group settings. It depends on the mindset of the teacher, but you might notice a distinct bias with the NCT towards natural birth and breastfeeding.

Antenatal classes are a great place to meet people in the same boat as you. *Most* new mums (and it's not compulsory – some are happy to go it alone) find that knowing and being in touch with at least one other woman in the same situation is a vital aid to sanity in the weeks and months after birth.

Pocket tip ☞

If you're not signed up to classes and you're worried about missing out on the social aspect, try and make a few more in advance of the birth, perhaps by logging on to an online community such as Netmums.

🚼 WHAT TO BUY FOR YOUR BABY 🚼

At this stage, the answer is 'not much'. You don't actually need more than a few basics to start out with. Most people also find that they get lots of clothes as gifts. However, make sure your newborn has:

- Something to wear
- Something to sleep on
- Something to be carried in

Pocket tip ☞

It makes sense to get the basics in with plenty of time to spare, just in case you have a premature arrival.

Your baby's basic needs at the start are:

- Up to 10 vests and the same number of sleepsuits. Your priorities are: comfort and something that is easily removable

- A cardigan for colder weather (perhaps two so you've always got one clean)

- A coat or jacket, unless it's a very warm time of year

- A hat (ditto)

- Lots of teeny-tiny nappies – disposables are the most convenient, but if the environment's a concern for you, and you can face the laundry issues, think about reusables. You'll also need a job lot of cotton wool; and some barrier or nappy cream

- A cot or moses basket

A moses basket

The basket is a nice idea because it's cosier for a tiny baby and you can move it from room to room, which, since they sleep so much when they're tiny, is very useful. However, your baby will only fit in it for three to five months, tops, and so they're not very economical. Most people borrow one – but for safety reasons, it's recommended that you always buy a new mattress.

- Bedding for the cot/basket – sheets are easier if they're fitted. Get quite a few in as they get very milk-soiled. You'll need one to two blankets depending on the time of year and these should be lightweight

- Muslins – once the baby's born you'll probably be walking around with one permanently draped over your shoulder, to mop up the sick, milk, etc

- A car seat – buy new, or if you're taking on one that's second-hand, only accept from a good friend in case it's been damaged in an accident, which could compromise its effectiveness

- A pram and/or sling

> **Prams or slings?**
>
> *The baby market is full of prams. Take your time and try before you buy. Features to look for are:*
>
> - *how light/sturdy it is*
> - *how well it 'handles'*
> - *how easily it can be collapsed and put up*
> - *whether you've got enough room to store it at home*
>
> *Slings are a popular transportation option for very young babies because they're less hassle and less space-consuming than prams. They can also be useful if you need to get something done around the house, but your baby refuses to be put down.*

- Something to wash him in – a baby bath isn't really necessary because you can just use a large, clean washing up bowl until he's a little older and can be safely held in the big bath. However, a baby bath on a stand, or one that fits over the main bath, is a godsend if you have a bad back.

Pocket tip 🍵

Baby toiletries really aren't necessary for a newborn; in fact, their delicate skin could well do without it.

🚼 WILL YOU NEED HELP? 🚼

If you both work, if you're a single parent, if you're expecting twins or more, if you're disabled or have other responsibilities such as elderly relatives to care for, now's the time to consider whether you need some help after the birth. You'll need to consider what will suit you and your family, as well as the cost implications. Here are some of your options, and the pros and cons of them.

RELATIVES

Pros	Cons
You have help from someone who is part of the baby's family and who you can trust.	It would be hard to terminate the arrangement if things don't work out without people getting upset.
It's usually free (or very inexpensive).	You may feel you're taking advantage of your relatives and may not relax as much as you should.
Your relative will probably relish the time with the baby and therefore may be flexible about hours worked.	It could be hard to get childcare over the hours you want without a rigid contract, and you might feel like you are asking too much.

PART-TIME HELP

Pros	Cons
You have regular help at the time – and in the way – you want it.	It will cost you, though how much depends on how many hours you want them to work.
If there are problems, or if your helper doesn't work out, it's much easier to resolve professionally than the stress of having to tell, say, your mother-in-law that it's not working out.	If they're off sick and you rely on them a lot, you could be stuck.
	They may not be flexible if you want them to do extra hours for some reason, and this can leave you in the lurch.

FULL-TIME HELP

Pros	Cons
You will get a lot of help.	This is the most expensive choice.
You have a professional relationship, so sorting out problems is easier than with a helper who is also part of your family.	They will need time off. It's a tough job and they are unlikely to be flexible about working extra hours.
	Some people feel uncomfortable having someone else living in the house permanently.

🍼 PACKING YOUR HOSPITAL BAG 🍼

You'll need to get together a bag for your hospital stay and keep it by the door, at least a couple of weeks before your due date. Assuming things go without complication, you probably won't stay in hospital for longer than a day and night. However short your visit turns out to be, though, you're going to need a certain amount of stuff to see you through labour and birth, and afterwards.

Pocket fact 🎲

The eggs of rabbits, gorillas, dogs, pigs, whales, mice and humans are all the same size.

WHAT TO PACK

- **Something to give birth in:** Although most hospitals will provide a gown, you might feel more comfortable in something of your own. Make sure it's something you're happy to throw away afterwards – an old, baggy t-shirt is ideal.

- **Maternity towels:** These are not the same as ordinary sanitary towels – they're bigger, and more absorbent – so make sure you get the right ones for the job. You may also get through rather more than you imagined – so stock up with several boxes, and take at least one to hospital in case you have to stay a while.

- **Big pants:** You'll need (and will want) some comfy knickers to fit your big sanitary towels in. Take at least six pairs, as you'll probably be changing them frequently.

- **Nursing bra and breast pads:** Try to get measured for a bra as near to your due date as possible – but bear in mind you might also need one in a size up, as your boobs will get even bigger when your milk comes two to three days after the birth.

If you don't intend to breastfeed, bottles and formula will usually be provided by the hospital (but obviously you'll need a good supply plus a steriliser and bottles at home).

- **A front-opening nightie or two:** You'll want something nicer to slip into after the birth, and a front-opener's ideal for breastfeeding.

- **Comfy clothing to change into before leaving:** Every bit of you will ache. A loose, soft tracksuit is what you need.

- **Toothbrush and toothpaste, and some basic toiletries:** There probably won't be anything in the hospital and one thing you're almost certain to want afterwards is a shower.

- **Hairbrush and makeup:** Someone's bound to want to take pictures of you before you've left hospital and, chances are, you won't be looking your best.

- **Warm socks and/or slippers:** Hospital floors can be pretty cold. Some women also like to keep socks on during labour, as your feet tend to be exposed.

- **Snacks and drinks:** Catering can be a hit and miss affair in maternity units, especially if you become hungry or thirsty in the middle of the night, so bring your own sustenance. Have something non-perishable in your suitcase like crackers or cereal bars, and pop in fresh stuff like fruit just before you leave. Don't forget some cartons of juice or bottles of water, too.

- **Boredom busters:** Labour can be a long, drawn-out affair. Take a good book, some magazines or music.

- **A camera.**

- **Your mobile phone:** Remember that hospitals generally have rules about turning mobiles off, though. You may also want to make sure you've got change for a payphone in case you can't get a signal.

- **Lip balm; sponge; water spray; stereo and your delivery music of choice:** All optional extras.

- **What you'll need for your baby:** Several soft cotton sleepsuits and vests; a cardigan or jacket; a hat (depending on the weather); a blanket for the journey home; nappies; and cotton wool. Most important of all is the car seat: unless you're walking home, the hospital won't let you leave without one of these. You can get lots of useful advice about car seats and car safety from the Child Accident Prevention Trust (www.capt.org.uk).

🛒 NAMING YOUR BABY 🛒

HOW TO CHOOSE A NAME

Choosing your baby's name is something most parents really look forward to – whether you know the sex or not.

> *Pocket fact* 🎲
>
> *The average length of a name is six letters.*

Top tips

- **Fall in love with the name(s) you've chosen:** Make sure you pick a name that makes you smile because, if you love it, hopefully your child will too.

- **Don't listen to other people:** If you've fallen in love with a name that's slightly unusual or bucks tradition, keep quiet about your choice until the baby's born – people won't criticise a named baby.

- **Research:**

  o Get a baby name book and flick through at your leisure.

  o Go on the internet and check out the statistics for how common the names you like are – will there be 10 Emmas in your daughter's class?

  o Make lists of names you hear during the run-up to the birth.

- **Find a name with meaning:** They may just be inspired to live up to their name.

- **Have fun:** Laughing at the ones you'd never dream of choosing can really help you narrow it down to the ones you would.

- **Expand your mind:** don't rule out the weird ones just yet! Some quirky names can work really well – see below.

> *Pocket fact* 🔡
>
> *The shortest names are only two letters long (Al, Ed, Jo and Ty), but the longest could be any length imaginable. Popular 11-letter names include Bartholomew, Christopher, Constantine and Maximillian.*

- **Try it out:** While you're pregnant, talk to your baby and address him using a variety of your favourite names to see if he responds.

- **What if you can't agree?** Research a number of names you and your partner are both interested in and make a point of discussing your reasons for liking or disliking them. Avoid sticking to your guns on a name one of you really isn't happy with. Try compromising and picking two middle names so you both have a name in there you love. It is important that you both eventually agree on the name you are giving your baby, even if it means losing out on that one you've had your heart set on for a while.

Top 10 Baby Boy Names	Top 10 Baby Girl Names
1. Jack	1. Ruby
2. Oliver	2. Olivia
3. Charlie	3. Jessica
4. Alfie	4. Grace
5. Harry	5. Sophie
6. Thomas	6. Emily
7. James	7. Chloe
8. Joshua	8. Lily
9. William	9. Amelia
10. Daniel	10. Evie

THINK TO THE FUTURE

- Will the name you've chosen stand the test of time?

- Will they be able to confidently enter a room and give a crucial business presentation with an awkward or unpronounceable name?

- Even on a smaller scale, can they survive the potential minefields of primary and secondary school with a name that could be easily shortened to something embarrassing?

- Would you want to try catching criminals as Police Officer Apple Blossom? You don't want to give your child a name that they just cannot live with for the rest of their lives, so make your choice based on what's appropriate for an adult as well as a child.

New Zealand law prevents parents from giving their children names that would cause offence or are more than 100 characters long.

Banned names
The following names were all banned by registration officials in New Zealand:
Cinderella Beauty Blossom
Fat Boy
Fish and Chips (twins)
Sex Fruit
Stallion
Talula Does The Hula From Hawaii
Yeah Detroit

Allowed names
These names, however, were all permitted by the same officials:
All Blacks
Benson and Hedges (twins)
Ford Mustang
Kaos
Midnight Chardonnay
Number 16 Bus Shelter
Superman (changed from 4real)
Violence

NICKNAMES

- Nicknames can range from the common – Mike from Michael, Sam from Samantha – to the trendy, funny or downright insulting. Many Richards refuse to be called 'Dick' and Francescas prefer 'Fran' over 'Fanny'.

- A way to avoid embarrassing nicknames is to select one for your child that you actually like so that others don't even get a mention. Call your daughter Elizabeth by Liz, Lizzie or Libby if you don't like Betty or Beth, and no one will even consider the alternatives.

- Pre-empt problem nicknames by saying the name you've chosen out loud and trying to find rhymes for it.

Pocket fact 🎲

A Chinese couple were prevented from naming their child '@' in 2007, despite their reasoning that it was simply a modern choice of name in this technological age.

INITIALS

- Does the first letter of your baby's surname's lend itself easily to amusing acronyms, and would choosing certain forenames only exacerbate the problem?

- Across the UK, there are people whose initials spell out three letter words – from RAT and FAG to FAB or POP (some are better than others, so do check!).

Amusing initials

- Earl E Bird
- I P Freely
- Al E Gador
- S Lugg
- Warren T
- IC Blood

Amusing acronyms of real people

- Samuel Alan Spencer – SAS

- Neil Christopher Parker – NCP (the car park)

- Jake Clive Baxter – JCB

- Patricia Mary Simpson – PMS

- David Vernon Durante – DVD

- George Barry Holmes – GBH

YOUR SURNAME

Try to avoid forenames that might lead to unfortunate phrases when combined with certain surnames to prevent a lifetime of embarrassment for your child. Write down all the names you like alongside your child's last name and have someone else read them out loud.

Unfortunate forename/surname combinations

- Barb Dwyer

- Ben Dover

- Duane Pipe

- Harry Rump

- Isabella Horn

- Jenny Taylor

- Justin Time

- Mary Christmas

- Russell Sprout

- Stan Still

SPOONERISMS

Be careful also of spoonerisms – where the first letters or syllables get swapped around to form new words.

An unfortunate and recent example of this would be Angelina Jolie and Brad Pitt's daughter Shiloh, whom they named Shiloh Jolie-Pitt to avoid the inevitable Shiloh Pitt spoonerism. Try to avoid making the same mistake!

Famous name spoonerisms

- Mike Baker (bike maker)

- Shirley Bassey (burly chassis)

- Kelly Brook (belly crook)

- Clive James (jive claims)

- Gene Kelly (keen jelly)

- Sarah Palin (para sailing)

- Shiloh Pitt (pile o' s***)

QUIRKY NAMES

Many parents shy away from quirky names as they are very aware of potential ridicule in the playground or of the name dating quickly. However, a quirky name should not be dismissed too soon:

- It is not true that babies are as influenced by their names as people believe. There is no scientific evidence to say that names dictate who we become, which means that you cannot give your child a perfect or imperfect name, whichever one you finally pick.

- Your child's name will never be forgotten by other people.

- A quirky name often requires a quirky personality. Will your genes produce the personality to match?

SPELLINGS AND PRONUNCIATION

Some parents take great joy in experimenting with unusual variations of traditional names, while others prefer names to be instantly recognisable.

- Try to avoid making a common name too long or too unusual in its spelling because this will be the first thing your child learns how to write. They will also be subjected to constant corrections during their lifetime as other people misspell or mispronounce their name in ever more frustrating patterns.

- Make sure the name isn't too long to fit on forms or name badges because they'll simply stop using it and take on a nickname instead.

- Substituting the odd 'i' for a 'y' isn't too bad, but turning the name Jonathan into Jonnaythanne doesn't do anyone any favours.

Britain has seen an increase in 'text' language spellings

An	*Jaicub*
Camron	*Jayk*
Conna	*Lora*
Ema	*Patryk*
Esta	*Samiul*
Flicity	*Summa*
Helin	

MIDDLE NAMES

Names from the family tree

- If you know you or your partner is related to Charles Darwin, you might choose Charles or even Darwin as a middle name for your son, or if your great-great-grandmother had a particularly unusual name and supported the suffragette movement, you could choose her name for your daughter's middle name.

- If a relative passed away recently you could choose their name as a way of honouring their memory, or you could even choose it while they're still alive to make them proud.

- It is becoming more and more common to give a parent's first name as a middle name to newborns.

Unusual names

Along with a wider variety of first names in recent years, parents are choosing more unusual middle names too. As middle names are used far less frequently, this is an opportunity for parents to have an unusual name included that they wouldn't perhaps use otherwise.

Pocket fact

At 4–8 weeks a baby starts to smile socially.

Common names

Many people choose a nice traditional middle name: for girls Anne, Marie, May and Rose are all popular, as are Andrew, David, James and Thomas for boys.

Amusing middle name combinations

Blanche Kerr Tane (blanche curtain)
Claire May Dye (Claire may die)
Harry Armand Bach (hairy arm and back)
Justin Miles North (just ten miles north)
Laura Lynne Hardy (Laurel and Hardy)
Liz May Read (Liz may read)
Mary Annette Woodin (marionette wooden)
Norma Leigh Lucid (normally lucid)
May Ann Naze (mayonnaise)
Sam Ann Fisher (salmon fisher)

Multiple middle names

It is becoming more and more common to have several middle names, particularly if parents like more than one or want to include a family name as well. Be careful not to have too many, though, as this makes life very difficult when filling out official forms or enrolling your child in school.

The longest name in the world

The Glastonbury teenager named **Captain Fantastic Faster Than Superman Spiderman Batman Wolverine Hulk And The Flash Combined** *changed his* *name from George Garratt in 2008. He claims to have the longest name in the world. If he does then he replaces Texan woman **Rhoshandiatellyneshiaunneveshenk Koyaanisquatsiuth Williams**, whose 57-letter length name pales in comparison to Captain's 81.*

🛒 THINGS TO DO BEFORE 🛒 YOUR BABY IS BORN

- Have a good tidy up, but don't obsess about the skirting boards and a designer nursery. There's more important stuff to do.

- Do a big shop of basics such as loo roll and staple foods, so you don't have to worry about shopping once you've brought your baby home.

- Make meals for the freezer if you're that way inclined.

- Get lots of sleep – while you still can . . .

- Do some research into birth and think about how you hope yours might pan out.

- Read up on baby care. Lots of new mums realise they were so busy reading about pregnancy and birth, they forgot to work out how to look after their baby.

- Go out – for a meal, to the cinema. When your baby is born, your social life will die.

- Go for a 'babymoon' with your partner. Whether a proper holiday or a relaxing mini-break, it's a great idea to get away with your other half for a while.

- Start thinking about baby names – even if you can't quite decide, you'll have a few to choose from when you see your baby.

- They say it's a good idea to have your hair cut into an 'easy to maintain' style since you won't have time to go the hairdressers once your baby is born. Although slightly depressing, this is probably true.

- Practise some relaxation and breathing techniques and some birthing positions. If you're hoping your birth partner will be on hand with a bit of pain relieving massage, get him (or her) to have a trial run.

- Pack your hospital bag. It's a good idea to have this by the door ready to go at least a couple of weeks before your due date.

👶 YOUR FINAL CHECKLIST 👶

- Pack your bag and your birth plan, if you have one.

- Have your maternity notes ready if you've been keeping them at home.

- Make sure the house is reasonably shipshape and that you've got a bit of food in the freezer.

- Make sure the car works and has always got petrol in it (this one's for him).

- Put your birth partner/person responsible for transporting you to hospital on red alert (hint: they'll need to stay sober so they can drive at short notice, and they need to always be at the other end of their mobile).

- Have numbers for your midwife/maternity unit in a prominent place.

- Have a car seat and the few basics your baby will need ready.

8

THE BIRTH

There's enough information about what goes on during labour that you could write a whole book on it. Here, we give you a whistle-stop tour through the stages and answer possible questions you might have. Tip – read this well before your due date to get familiar with what might happen!

🍼 NATURAL WAYS TO ENCOURAGE 🍼 LABOUR

There are various things that are said to bring on labour – remember, the only evidence that any of them work is anecdotal rather than scientific.

- **A hot curry:** If it works, it's probably something to do with a laxative effect that stimulates the uterus as well as the bowel but, really, there's no scientific evidence that this works. Don't attempt to have a really hot one if you're not used to it.

- **Sex:** The theory *is* based in scientific evidence, since sperm contains prostaglandins, which are said to soften the cervix, and the hormone oxytocin – which stimulates contractions – is released when a woman orgasms.

- **Nipple touching:** Stimulation of the boobs aids the release of oxytocin, as when you orgasm. The idea is to use your palm and rub both nipple and areola (the dark skin surrounding the nipple) in a circular motion. It's reckoned that you need to do this for an hour three times a day if it's actually going to work.

- **Pineapple:** This contains the enzyme bromelain, which is said to boost production of prostaglandins. You have to eat it in large quantities to get enough enzymes to be effective.

- **Reflexology, aromatherapy, homeopathy and acupuncture:** Practitioners of all these alternative therapies claim they might give a natural kick-start to labour. There's no science to back this, but it's worth a try if you've got an open mind.

- **Long walks:** Moving around and keeping upright could help for the simple reason that gravity might jiggle your baby further down towards your cervix.

Don't try . . .

Raspberry leaf tea: *Although this might be helpful in preparing the uterus for birth if taken in the last month or two (but no earlier) of pregnancy, it's a myth that a single dose or cup will trigger labour.*

Castor oil: *An old wives' favourite, and another method based on bowel stimulation, but not really to be recommended, as castor oil tastes foul and could leave you nauseous, dehydrated and suffering from diarrhoea and painful bowel cramps.*

ENGAGEMENT

At some point from around 37 weeks, and sometimes earlier for a first baby, your baby's head will 'engage' – in other words, the baby drops down into your pelvis in readiness for birth.

> *Pocket fact*
>
> *The average child shares their birthday with 9 million people.*

WHEN YOU'RE NEARLY THERE (BUT NOT QUITE)

Your body may start to gear itself up for labour for a few days or even weeks before labour. The following signs are useful indicators, but there'll usually be no need to panic.

- **More vaginal discharge:** It's normal to have some throughout pregnancy, but towards the end it can increase, caused by the baby's head pressing on the cervix.
- **Backache**, or a period-pain-like feeling.
- **A 'show':** This is when the jelly-like plug (it looks like heavy discharge, and will often be streaked with blood) that seals the cervix comes away. It can do this some days or even a couple of weeks in advance of labour beginning, or it may not happen until the last minute.
- **Stronger Braxton Hicks:** 'Practice' contractions actually occur for a long time before your due date – they don't always become noticeable until later and can become really quite intense, and uncomfortable even, in the final few weeks. Lots of first-timers wonder if the Braxton Hicks they're experiencing are real contractions.

- **A bout of diarrhoea:** This can happen sometimes about 24 hours before the birth, clearing the bowels in readiness for labour.

Pocket fact 🔡

The most popular day of the week to give birth is Tuesday.

'If pregnancy were a book they would cut the last two chapters.'
Nora Ephron

🛒 YOUR WATERS BREAK 🛒

At some point, the sack of amniotic fluid surrounding your baby will burst and spurt or drizzle out from your vagina – this is your waters breaking, although the technical term is spontaneous rupture of the membrane (SROM).

For most women, this doesn't happen until after contractions have begun and labour has started. However, for about 1 woman in 20 women, waters break before labour starts (it's known then as prelabour rupture of the membranes, or PROM).

Pocket tip 🥢

If your waters go but your contractions haven't yet begun, it's a sure sign that they soon will. You should give your maternity unit or midwife a call if it happens to you. You'll probably be asked to go in for an assessment because, once your waters go, there's an increased risk of infection.

In 9 out of 10 cases, labour starts within 24 hours of waters breaking early. If it goes beyond that, an induction will probably be recommended as the infection risk will continue to increase.

🛒 CONTRACTIONS 🛒

The start of proper contractions means the first stage of labour is under way. Contractions are almost always mild to start with and spaced far apart – perhaps every 20 minutes. This stage, known as the latent phase, can go on for ages – a whole day or even two is not unusual, particularly in a first birth.

Pocket fact 🎲

Contractions – also known as labour pains – are what happen when the muscles of the uterus flex as it works to open up the cervix (the neck of the womb), from where your baby will soon be making his exit.

What to do during contractions

- It's a good idea to stay upright and active if it happens during the day, and to try to sleep or doze if it's night-time.

- Try to have something to eat and drink, too, if you can, to boost your strength – although admittedly some women do feel off their food around now (and sometimes, even, feel sick or vomit during this phase).

- This is also a good time to have a bath, to help you relax and which may also soothe the pain of the contractions.

- Other ways to pass the time in as relaxing a way as possible include going for a gentle walk, or watching something you love on telly, listening to your favourite music, and getting your other half to give you a massage.

What if my baby's coming RIGHT NOW?

- *Try to call someone who can be with you quickly.*
- *Ring the emergency number on your notes. If you can't find the number, dial 999 and ask for an ambulance. Make sure the front door's open so they can all get in.*
- *Try to find some towels — one to save your carpet and a large clean one to wrap your baby in.*
- *Kneel with your head on your forearms and keep your bottom as high up in the air as possible. Resist pushing if you can. Try breathing in a pattern of three short pants and a long blow. This can help delay things a bit.*
- *If you can't resist the urge to push and your baby starts to make its way out before anyone's got to you, don't panic. Hold on to him, and carefully check to make sure the cord isn't looped round his neck (ease it gently back over if it is, but don't pull it).*
- *Once your baby's all the way out, wrap him up to keep him warm. There might be mucus or fluids in his nose preventing him from breathing properly, which you can push out by stroking down the sides of his nose.*
- *Place the baby on his front across your belly with his head lower than his body to allow any remaining fluid to drain out, and firmly rub his back with the towel.*
- *Don't pull on the cord, and don't attempt to cut it — the professional who comes to your aid will sort that for you, but do cuddle him close and try putting him to your breast. Your placenta should follow soon afterwards, still attached to the cord.*

🛏 'ESTABLISHED' LABOUR 🛏

Eventually the contractions will begin to come more often, be longer-lasting, and feel more intense.

- Once they're coming thick and fast, about every four to five minutes, you're considered to be in 'established' or 'active' labour.

- Even now, you're likely to be between 6 and 12 hours away from having your baby. Generally, midwives encourage women to stay at home for as long as they can before coming in to hospital, assuming there are no problems.

- Make a call to the unit once your contractions are coming regularly, every five to six minutes or so. You could then be advised by the duty midwife to come in, or you may be advised to stay put a while.

Pocket fact 🎲

An average labour for the first-time mum is said to be 12 hours. Second labours are often shorter than your first – but this isn't guaranteed!

'Fully dilated'

At the hospital, the midwife will measure your cervix. If you're '1cm dilated' you've got a way to go. Labour isn't considered to be established until the cervix is 3–4cm dilated, and you're not 'fully dilated' and ready to go until it opens up to 10cm.

What your birth partner can do for you during labour and delivery

- Keep you entertained (or just provide company) if you're enduring a long, boring wait for action.

- Massage your back to help ease the pain.

- Fetch you snacks, drinks or anything else you need.

- Help keep you cool by sponging or spraying your face.

- Offer words of encouragement and support.

- Speak up or ask questions if something's happening you're not keen on or sure about (but only if you give them the nod first . . .).

- Provide support if you want to give birth kneeling, squatting or standing up.

- Let you know all's going well from his vantage point down 'the business end'.

Pocket fact 🎲

Some women in history have been known to be in labour for up to 3 weeks. The birth of Christ in historical writings is said to have lasted 7 weeks 4 days.

🍼 HERE COMES YOUR BABY 🍼

As your baby's head moves right down through the cervix towards the vagina, you might feel an overwhelming urge to push (referred to as 'bearing down') but if it's not yet time to do so, because the cervix isn't fully dilated, your midwife will ask you to hold back.

Pocket tip 🖢

Help counter the urge to push by breathing in short puffs, or pants.

Your midwife will guide you with each contraction, she will urge you to stop or slow your pushing, breathing out in puffs.

Once the baby's head is out, the hard work is done: you should only need to give another push to get the body out.

Sometimes, in spite of your best efforts, your baby won't budge. When this happens, your doctor might suggest using forceps or vacuum extraction (Ventouse) to help him out (see below).

Pocket fact 🔡

Giraffes are born with the mother standing up, on the lookout for predators. That means a long drop of 5 to 7 feet to the ground – long enough to break the baby's umbilical cord.

🛒 ONCE YOUR BABY IS BORN 🛒

- The midwife will quickly look over him and check his breathing, skin colour, heart rate, muscle tone and reflex response. Occasionally, a baby will need his passages suctioned and sometimes a little extra oxygen, in order to help him breathe.

- She'll then clean him up a bit, before handing him over for a cuddle.

Pocket tip 🥄

Don't be surprised if your baby looks kind of hideous. As well as being rather slimy, newborns can be hairy, blotchy, somewhat swollen, squinty-eyed, and pointy-headed. Luckily, he'll be beautiful to you.

- Meanwhile, the umbilical cord will be clamped and cut and, if you need stitches, you'll get them.

- You may feel high as a kite at this point, or you may feel drained and slightly depressed. Either is normal.

Pocket fact 🔠

Your baby is born with very sophisticated hearing and can work out where a sound is coming from just 10 minutes after being born. Psychologists have found that babies as young as just 2 days old can recognise their mothers from a tape recording of only one syllable.

🍼 DELIVERY OF THE PLACENTA 🍼

Contractions (milder ones) will continue as your body prepares to expel the placenta. This process should happen naturally within an hour or so of birth (and if you're keen for a natural delivery of the placenta, it's something you could put in your birth plan); however, it's common these days to be given an injection to speed things up.

Placenta trivia

- *In the UK, most women leave their placentas at the hospital for them to dispose of it. In other cultures, it plays an important role.*
- *In New Zealand, Maori culture is to bury the placenta, to signify the relationship between humans and earth.*
- *The Navajo Indians of the USA also bury the placenta and umbilical cord in a sacred site, especially if the baby dies during birth.*
- *In Cambodia and Costa Rica, they bury the placenta to ensure the health of the baby and the mother.*
- *The Kwakiutl of British Columbia bury girls' placentas to give the girl skill in digging clams, and expose boys' placentas to ravens to encourage future prophetic visions.*
- *In Turkey, the placenta and umbilical cord must be disposed of properly to make sure the child is devout in later life.*
- *Native Hawaiians believe that the placenta is a part of the baby and will plant it with a tree, which then grows with the child.*
- *In some cultures, the placenta is eaten; this is known as placentophagy.*

🛒 ASSISTED DELIVERY 🛒

If your baby is having trouble, or if you are too exhausted to push, you may have an assisted delivery. Here the obstetrician will use either forceps or a vacuum extractor (Ventouse) to get hold of your baby and ease him out.

- **Forceps** are curved tongs that look a bit like a large pair of salad servers. If these are used, you'll need to have an episiotomy (see below) to allow room for the forceps to be inserted and fit round your baby's head.

- A **Ventouse** or **vacuum extractor** is more like a sink plunger: it has a plastic or metal cap which fixes to your baby's head, and a vacuum pump which is used to cause a suction effect. Vacuum extraction is more common and is a gentler option as it doesn't usually require an episiotomy and you're less likely to suffer any damage or pain as a consequence.

- In either case, you'll need to lie on your back and have your feet placed in stirrups. You'll also need pain relief in the form of a local anaesthetic or epidural.

- If it doesn't work, the obstetrician will suggest a Caesarean section.

- You're well within your rights to question your doctor if he decides you'll need intervention, and some people believe it's not always needed when suggested – but do remember the doctor does have your baby's and your well-being in mind.

EPISIOTOMY

- This is a cut of the perineum and vagina, performed by a mid-wife or doctor when considered necessary to help your baby make his exit.

- You'll be given an effective form of pain relief in the form of a local anaesthetic injection (unless you've already got an epidural in place).

You'll need to be stitched up again afterwards (as indeed you may be if you tear naturally) and unfortunately this can cause much discomfort after the birth. It should only take a month for stitches to heal completely.

🍼 WHEN YOU NEED AN EMERGENCY 🍼 CAESAREAN SECTION

Sometimes in a labour that has started off normally, an obstetrician may decide that the fastest and safest way to get your baby out is by performing a Caesarean section (c-section). Read this section to calm your fears, or answer any questions about them – ahead of time. One will probably be mooted if:

- You suddenly develop pre-eclampsia (see p. 56).

- Your labour isn't progressing and you're getting exhausted, or your baby has become stuck or distressed.

- Your baby isn't getting the oxygen he needs, or his heartbeat has become irregular.

- A potentially dangerous complication, such as placental abruption (see p. 63) has occurred.

What happens in a c-section

- Once you've given consent for a Caesarean to be carried out, you'll be given an anaesthetic.

- You'll also need a catheter and a drip in your hand, to administer fluids or pain relief when needed.

- Once the anaesthetic's kicked in, an incision is made, usually horizontally across the lower part of the abdomen at the top of the pubic bone or 'bikini line'. This all takes place behind a screen.

- A second cut is then made in the uterus so the baby can be lifted out. The baby will be handed straight to a paediatrician (who will have been invited along as a matter of routine) to be checked.

● If he's very small, or poorly, your baby will have to go straight to the special care unit. If not, he can be handed to your birth partner or carefully placed next to you for a cuddle whilst you're stitched up.

Recovery after a c-section

● *You should have got over the worst after six weeks, but some women say they still don't feel right for up to a year afterwards.*

● *You'll have to stay in hospital for three to four days, on average, and you'll need some heavy-duty painkilling medication.*

● *You'll probably find even simple activities like sitting up and walking hard work, and will need lots of help and support in doing so.*

● *There's no reason why you can't cuddle and breastfeed your baby.*

● *You'll see a physiotherapist in hospital who will help you to get walking and show you some exercises to do.*

● *Don't panic if your incision site looks very obvious or vivid at this point — it will shrink and fade to a fine, pale line with time.*

● *You'll be warned not to drive for at least a couple of weeks after having a c-section and to avoid lifting anything heavy for several months.*

🚼 WHAT HAPPENS IF YOU GO 🚼 PAST YOUR DUE DATE?

Normal pregnancies can continue for up to 43 weeks, so it's not unusual for women to go past their due date.

- If there's no sign of your baby by your due date, you'll usually be offered a 'membrane sweep' – your midwife or doctor will run a finger around the inner edge of your cervix to encourage it to start dilating.

- If this doesn't work, you'll usually be offered a day in the next week to have your labour induced. Most doctors will be keen for this to happen within 14 days of your due date – even if your pregnancy has been normal and there are no other risk factors.

INDUCTION

About one in five women in this country are induced. If an induction is suggested, you should be given a full explanation as to why, as well as what the risks, benefits and alternatives are, and given time to think about and discuss it before making a decision. You should still be offered the chance to wait for labour to start naturally if you prefer.

Induction could mean a very abrupt and intense start to labour pains (you may need to consider an epidural).

👶 AFTER THE BIRTH 👶

Some time soon after you've had your baby – assuming he's well and doesn't need special care – you'll both be taken to a post-natal ward. You may want to sleep, but you may still be buzzing and want to spend some time holding, or just staring at, your baby.

Assuming you had an uncomplicated vaginal delivery, you'll probably be dispatched from the maternity unit within about 12 hours of the birth.

9

THE FIRST FEW WEEKS

🍼 TRANSPORTING YOUR 🍼
BABY HOME

- Remember that you won't be allowed to take your baby home in your car if you do not have a correctly sized baby seat fitted and ready for action.

- Make sure your baby is wrapped up adequately if it's a cold day – even if you think it's mild, your newborn will be very sensitive to temperature changes. Put him in a hat, babygrow and a light blanket. Add mittens and a warm coat in winter.

- Don't take your baby out of the car seat during the journey – even if he cries a lot.

Newborn babies: the surprising facts

- *His first poos are dark and sticky. The dark sticky stuff will soon give way to something yellow or green and runny (in breastfed babies) but paler and firmer (and generally smellier) if formula-fed.*
- *His skin is very often flaky, blotchy, rashy or spotty. (Check with your health visitor if you're worried, but in most cases it will be harmless and normal.)*

- *He may be very hairy. This is the remains of lanugo, the covering that protected him in the womb, and will drop out soon.*
- *He may also still have vernix on him and so be a bit greasy. Don't bother trying to wash it off, it'll help protect against dry skin.*
- *His head may be a weird shape, squished by the journey down the birth canal (and especially if vacuum extraction or forceps were used to ease him out). The soft spot on the top, where the skull bones have yet to fuse, is called the fontanelle. It's likely to be a year or more before it closes up.*
- *His eyes may squint. This is because the muscles around them have yet to develop.*
- *The remains of the umbilical cord stays attached to his belly for a few weeks after birth, after which it shrivels and drops off. Let your midwife or health visitor know if it looks sore, as it can sometimes become infected.*
- *He may sleep for hours and hours on end during the day in the first few weeks. Make the most of the time to catch up on some rest yourself!*
- *Your baby is born with 300 separate bones. Some of these bones will fuse together, as adults have 206 bones.*
- *Your baby can breathe and swallow at the same time until 7 months, which an adult cannot.*
- *Babies are born without kneecaps.*

'A baby is something you carry inside you for nine months, in your arms for three years and in your heart till the day you die.'

Mary Mason

☕ FEEDING YOUR BABY ☕

Getting enough nourishment down your new charge is going to be one of your primary preoccupations over the coming weeks and months.

BREASTFEEDING

Equipment

- Breast pads
- Nipple cream for sore nipples – midwives usually recommend Lansinoh, which is made from a pure form of lanolin
- Easy-opening breastfeeding bras and a selection of tops that either lift easily or unfasten down the front
- Muslins to mop up spills and provide a little privacy
- A breast pump: useful a bit later on if you want to express your milk into a bottle so someone else can feed your baby – don't try this for the first four to six weeks, to allow yourself a good chance to get breastfeeding established

Pocket fact 🎲

Women have a quicker and more powerful physiological response to their baby crying than men do.

Pros

- Breasfeeding is natural, and therefore your milk will give your baby exactly all of the nutrients and hormones that it needs.
- You will both enjoy the physical closeness of breastfeeding.
- If your baby is in bed with you, you don't have to get out of bed to feed him in the night.

- It's incredibly convenient having milk constantly on tap regardless of when or where you are.

- Your breast comes fully sterilised – you don't have to clean and fill bottles.

Cons

- The baby will need to spend more time feeding since breast milk is less filling.

- Only the baby's mother can breastfeed the baby, so you can't delegate the job in the middle of the night or go out for a period of time because no one else can feed him.

- You may feel uncomfortable breastfeeding your baby in public.

- It can be difficult, frustrating and stressful to get the hang of breastfeeding.

- Sore nipples can make breastfeeding extremely painful, and there's a chance of mastitis, an infection of the breast.

Pocket tip ☞

Allow yourself plenty of time to adjust to having a baby in the house. It's a steep learning curve and one you need to take at a steady pace.

Tips for successful breastfeeding

- Make sure you're comfortable.

- Offer your baby the boob whenever he seems to want it. Although this can be exhausting, it's the best way to keep your supplies up – and it's not forever. Within a month or two, feeds will become speedier and more widely spaced.

- Let your baby drain the whole breast before offering the other – and go back to that one first at the next feed.

- Have lots of breast pads to hand because milk will leak out a lot early on.

- Don't introduce a bottle or dummy while you're getting breast-feeding established, in case your baby becomes confused.

- Keep *yourself* well fed and watered while you're breastfeeding. Breastfeeding mums need about 400 calories more a day than when they were pregnant.

BOTTLEFEEDING

As many a mum of a bouncing, bottle-fed baby will tell you, formula's a perfectly good alternative to breast milk, as long as you stick to the rules on hygiene and preparation.

Equipment

- A steriliser

- Bottles: these generally come with teats and lids, which you need to keep sterile

- Formula: make sure you get the right age range – you want the one for newborns, not 'follow-on-milk'

Pros

- It's easy to learn how to bottle feed.

- Anyone can bottle feed the baby.

- Father and baby get more chance to bond as he can take his turn bottle feeding.

- Although both hands are occupied, it is generally easier to bottle feed a baby on the move than to breastfeed it.

Cons

- Formula lacks some human hormones that are in breast milk.

- You have to get up in the night to sort out and warm the bottle.

- You need to spend time cleaning and sterilising, which can be a lot of work. If you travel, all this stuff has to go with you.

- You can prepare for a routine feed, but your baby might not abide by this. Sometimes you'll have to let him cry while you prepare the bottle.

Pocket tip ☕

If the weather is very hot, a formula-fed baby may need extra water. Boil it first to sterilise it, and then cool it down before giving it to the baby. Put it in a bottle just as you do the formula milk.

A BIT OF BOTH

Some mums who struggle to breastfeed exclusively find a happy compromise in mixed feeding – some breastfeeds, some formula. Your breasts will quickly adjust to the decreased demand, though, so if you do start this, you can't go back.

Pocket tip ☕

If you're in any doubt about something, remember you don't have to tackle it alone: put in a call to your midwife or health visitor (for more on the support services you'll be offered after birth, see below). If you can't get hold of someone quickly and you feel you need to, you can always call NHS Direct. It's a good idea to put all the important telephone numbers somewhere prominent, so you're not scrabbling around in a panic if you need them.

🛒 YOUR BODY 🛒

How you feel in the weeks after having a baby will depend on what kind of birth you had.

- **Bleeding:** Known as lochia, every woman has a postnatal discharge of blood, mucus and tissue as the womb sheds its lining. It will normally stop altogether within six weeks. You'll need plenty of maternity pads to cope with the flow.

- **Afterpains:** Your uterus has to contract back to its normal size in the days after birth and this can be painful, particularly whilst breastfeeding. Take paracetamol, or try a heat pack or hot water bottle.

- **Vagina and perineum:** If you tore or had an episiotomy you will be very sore, and if you didn't, you'll feel bruised and tender. Take painkillers and warm baths. Arnica will help relieve bruising and inflammation and boost the healing process. Doing your pelvic floor exercises will help healing, as it increases blood flow to the area.

- **Bowels:** Trying to do a poo in the days after birth can be difficult. Keep up your fibre intake and drink plenty of water. If necessary, ask your midwife to recommend a gentle laxative treatment.

- **Breasts:** A couple of days after birth, your milk 'comes in', and your breasts will become unbearably tender. It won't last longer than a couple of days. The best way to relieve the pain and pressure this causes is to feed your baby if you're breast-feeding. Let your midwife know if any red patches appear on your breast, and/or you're suffering from flu-like symptoms: this could be a sign of mastitis, a condition that causes the breast tissue to inflame painfully and may need treatment. If you're not breastfeeding, there'll be a painful few days whilst the milk subsides. You'll need a snug-fitting bra, and possibly some paracetamol, to ease your way through this period.

- **Belly:** Your tummy will be flabby. Don't worry about this – there'll be time enough in the future to get your shape back. As for stretch marks, if you have them, they'll fade eventually – although they won't go altogether.

- **Weak or leaky bladders:** This is a common consequence of giving birth. Do your pelvic floor exercises.

The people looking after you

- *In most areas you'll remain under the care of a community midwife for around 10 days, and she should drop in on you several times during this period to make sure both you and your baby are doing okay, after which your health visitor – a qualified nurse or midwife who works in the community with families – will take over.*

- *Your baby should get a full medical once-over within three days of his birth – this could either be when you're still in hospital, or once you get home, usually by a visiting GP. His height and weight measurements will be taken, and checks made on his eyes, heart, hips, and (boys only – naturally) his testes.*

- *Your midwife will want to make sure you're doing okay, too. She'll check your belly, any stitches and ask about your general health.*

- *Both you and your baby will also be offered a more comprehensive check-up, usually with a GP or practice nurse, six to eight weeks after birth.*

BABYCARE BASICS

Washing your baby: You can just 'top and tail' your newborn baby and you don't even need a baby bath for this, just a clean washing-up bowl of warm water. Undress him, wrap him in a towel to keep warm, and then gently wipe his eyes, face, neck and around the ears (not inside), around the cord stump, hands and nappy area. Watch out in particular for dribbles of milk gathering in folds under his neck and armpits. Dry him by gently patting with a towel.

Changing your baby: Put a new nappy on your baby straight away after he's done a poo, or whenever it's getting a bit soggy, to help prevent nappy rash. Clean and dry his bottom thoroughly (cotton wool and water's usually recommended, but alcohol-free baby wipes won't cause any harm), and apply a little barrier cream.

Holding your baby: It's normal to feel scared about this at first, since new babies are just so small and delicate. The most important thing to remember is to support his head, as he has no strength in his neck muscles for the first few months.

CONTINUOUS CRYING

Between one and three hours a day of wailing is quite normal – and very often, it's for no discernible reason.

Up to a fifth of babies suffer from 'excessive' crying, which is usually called colic. No one's really sure why exactly this happens, although there are plenty of theories – the most popular is that it's due to pain caused by an immature digestive system.

- If your baby's crying relentlessly, check he's not hungry, tired, in need of a feed, or poorly.
- If it's none of those things, then work your way through a list

of potential solutions: try holding, cuddling, jiggling, rocking, swinging, singing, going for a walk or a drive.

- There are various commercial preparations, such as Infacol, which are said to help with colic – these won't definitely help, but you may feel it's worth a shot.

- Check with your health visitor or GP if you have a problem with a relentlessly crying baby, as once in a while there'll be a medical reason for his distress.

- The good news about colic is that it almost always eases up by the time your baby is about three months old.

It's very normal to have feelings of anger and desperation sometimes if you have a baby who cries a lot. When you get to a point where you've reached the end of your tether, try to enlist help from someone else until you can feel calm again – or, if there's no one around, put your baby in his cot and leave the room for a few moments and take some deep breaths.

SAFE SLEEPING

- Put your baby to sleep on his back.

- Make up his bedding at the foot of the cot (so he can't wriggle down under his covers).

- Make sure he's not overdressed (a single vest and sleepsuit's fine), and the room isn't too hot (16–20°C is ideal.)

- Don't put too much bedding on – one blanket's usually enough.

- Don't fall asleep with your baby on a sofa or chair, and think carefully before having your baby in bed with you.

- Don't smoke near your baby – or anywhere in the house.

- Keep your baby's crib or cot in your room with you for the first six months.

SLEEPLESS NIGHTS . . .

When they're not feeding, new babies usually sleep. Unfortunately, they don't differentiate between night and day, so you can fully expect to be woken four or more times by a new baby wanting to eat. Things do settle down and night wakings will (usually) become less frequent over the coming months. And later still, when your baby is five or six months old, there are techniques that will help him sleep through the whole night

COMBATING TIREDNESS – WHAT CAN YOU DO?

The first few weeks of your baby's life will be utterly tiring, even if you've got a good sleeper. Here are some tips on how to minimise tiredness – as you can't get rid of it altogether unfortunately . . . sorry.

- Enlist the help of your partner/mother or mother–in–law/best friend/sibling to be on duty for a few hours every few days to give you some designated napping time.

- Don't be afraid to ask for help, and do take up people's offers.

- Make sure you are getting a balanced diet, with the right amounts of vitamins and nutrients. Eat healthy snacks regularly, as this will keep your energy up.

- Take some gentle exercise and get some fresh air. A short walk will re-energise you and get your blood pumping round your body, making you feel less tired.

BOND WITH YOUR BABY

It's not always love at first sight. Plenty of new mums look down at the baby they've just produced and feel pretty blank. Give yourself time – you'll almost certainly be flooded with feelings of love for him at some point, soon. If not, then you mustn't be afraid to talk to your midwife about it. It could be that you're suffering from postnatal depression and for that, you'll need some kind of help.

TAKE IT EASY

The greatest advice anyone can give you is to take it easy straight after you've had your baby. Leave the housework, the cooking, the shopping – and delegate!

Above all, spend this time getting to know your baby and make the most of this undeniably special period in your baby's life. And enjoy it, good luck.

'When you have children, you realise nothing else is important.'
Claudia Schiffer

INDEX